Cracks in Sacred Walls

Yael Shany

CRACKS IN SACRED WALLS

YAEL SHANY

To my three wonderful children who I love and cherish.

Acknowledgements

My thanks to my dear children who have been my most vital mentors all along, as well as to my life long friend Aki who has been like the harsh water smoothing the pebbles to silk and shine.

My thanks and acknowledgement to Dr. Nathan Barnes, my devoted and helpful editor who supported me through the process to bring this book out to my readers, and since English is not my mother tongue and writing is not my profession, Nathan had a rough work here to accomplish.

I also like to acknowledge Sister Paula—without her this book would never be created, and many of us would not get this vital teaching opportunity for our lifelong health.

From the Editor

When I first read these emails, I was inspired by Sister Paula's struggle with changing her unhealthy lifestyle to a healthy one using the homeopathic approach. Yael tenderly and patiently guides Sister Paula through the process of loving herself, taking the time to eat properly, and developing a joyful and emotionally enriching way of life.

This book is an intimate view into a relationship between two very different individuals who find encouragement and strength in each other, sharing in common the journey to better health. I hope that you experience the same inspiration and hope that I do when I read these letters.

Very Best,
Nathan J. Barnes, PhD
Fort Worth, TX

Contents

A Letter to the Reader

As you open this book you may be surprised to find that my intentions are more than simply revealing a list of email exchanges between myself, an atheist, anti-establishment advocate, freethinker, alternative medicine practitioner, astrologer, classic homeopathy practitioner and artist and Sister Paula, Italian Catholic 73-year-old nun who was diagnosed with "aggressive" breast cancer. Sister Paula dedicated her life to serving God when she was just eighteen years old. I, on the other hand, was raised in Israel by an atheist family who were German WW2 refugees who asked, "Where was God?"

These letters serve as an important platform for me to share with you a message of daring, challenging you to take a leap of faith and jump out of your box, rethink tradition, your upbringing, social rules and manners, and even question the idea of "this is the way to do it." We are all the image and creation of our background, childhood environment, and disciplines. Many of us do take a different route as we grow up. Some of us rebel and change direction from what we were taught, or as our ancestors' expectations of us have been. At the same time, many of us prefer to cling and walk the *traditional* paths believing, "This is what I grew up with," or "This is what I was raised to believe."

Sister Paula reflects for us not only extreme tradition and the 'blind' religious followers, but also the part in each of us that dares not to derail from the "this is the only way to do it" way of thinking. The information Sister Paula could and did access is the same we all get through many different media avenues, books, news, research, radio, TV, and the list goes on—we are constantly being bombarded with endless information. Sister Paula too was living in this era of open information and free access, so I wonder what gave her the strength to deny the reasons for her declining health? Was it her ability to block out all the eye-opening facts she received, or, her conviction to keep her religious vows at any and all costs? The fact that she was a very strong woman physically is clear by the hard work she was doing still at the age of seventy-plus. Was it peer pressure, fear of change or fear of God? As her need not to be considered as rebel, or maybe her oldest fear of taking responsibility for her own life she now faced for the first time being diagnosed with cancer?

Sister Paula represents a big crowd of 'religious believers' or 'establishment followers' and those who in the US vote for a government that rules through corruption rather than standing up and shouting out loud: "The king is naked." Many of us are still trapped in the need to be led and naively trust those leaders know what's best for us. We do believe that the establishment probably knows what is or should be the right and best for the people. We live in a democratic country but we give them that power to rule for us, make the 'right' decision for us, rather than thinking and decide for ourselves. We bend with an ancient fear of the 'higher power', and we dare to walk a different path, we may see every adversity in our lives as a clear punishment and result of our individual choices. And that is a heavy truth to bear, so often no change seems easier and no revision is more bearable.

When the Yom-Kippur War broke out October of 1973, I lived in a small school staff village in the southern part of Israel, where I was a physical education and athletics trainer. Some of the residents in that village (who were not part of the school staff) believed beyond a shadow of doubt that this war was God's punishment for people who were not observing Sabbath, not keeping strict Kosher kitchens, and worst of all, not fasting on Yom-Kippur. They got out of their little houses and yelled at us for our sinful conduct and were absolutely sure that war was because of us.

This kind of reaction is not unusual even in our highly educated society here in the US, where the majority of religious people will not skip Sunday church or the Sabbath to the synagogue or the Muslims, their services on Friday in their mosque. And still, they mix these rituals with an egg-laying bunny, menorahs or midnight shopping for Ramadan or Christmas. And all of these shifts in tradition are accrued, and more so, encouraged.

Here is the question: if the commercial world has taken the liberty to modify, twist, and adjust religious symbols and traditional customs to its benefit, so why can't the individual modify and adjust the religious symbols and beliefs to their present time and reality? By doing so, many of us will find that not only will we enjoy a more meaningful religious and spiritual experience untainted by commercialism, but also be free of old ways that we know are not the best ways and in turn, as in Sister Paula's case, even avoid damage to our health.

Like millions of other people, I am dairy and wheat intolerant. When asked why don't I eat those products I always say, "I don't eat anything that smiled, had a mother and eyes." I cannot see myself eating dead animals or food that is naturally intended to feed the offspring of any animal. I also do not consume commercially processed and manufactured products that some people consider food.

Considering all that, how could I sit at a Passover-Seder table and adhere to traditional Jewish culinary customs? As a freethinker and responsible individual, I have decided what is right and healthy for me to eat and drink in order to preserve my life as healthy as possible… and that does not include all the 'musts' of any religious order.

For example, if Sister Paula would have taken a little extra time to prepare healthier food and rest at night without feeling guilty for attending to her own needs and health requirements, would that mean that she was worshipping God less? Should she not have taken the responsibility for her life in her own hands, rather than placing her life in 'HIS' hands and her sisters' or the community's hands? Sister Paula struggled to find the sweet spot between her lifestyle and devotion to the church and the present, personal needs she was lacking in the face of death. The balance and the ability to change and adjust, living in accordance with nature, we all need to learn (post young childhood) by self-thinking, assuming responsibility, and not blindly follow anything or anyone.

Tradition is a beautiful and very vital part of our national and religious gatherings and congregations, but as we allow these traditions to be modified and enhanced commercially and for the sake of power and control in order to tie us even tighter to the things that have nothing more to do with religion or tradition than any other material, intangible, non-spiritual and even unethical purpose. These warped traditions serve only the religious leaders and authorities, commercial industry and enable their corrupted lifestyles alone. For example, are the orthodox Jews aware of the smugglers and black market business conducted in the name of tradition, like the sky rocketing prices of a Kiddush cup, a special Yakama, and Tallit and Tefilin? The high prices of the kosher foods just because it is labeled "supervised by the Rabbinate," which in most cases is a flat lie. If feeding the poor on Christmas night is right and holy, why do Christians not do it daily? Are those poor people and children rich the rest of the year? Why should we pour millions of dollars into the religious leaders fancy shamelessly luxurious lifestyle? I think that being true to ourselves, and to others—to those we serve, means that we should find the best ways as individuals that we might serve God. This means, 'serve your brother nature' and do not bow to hypocrisy and corruption.

We need to start thinking as educated, valued and respectful individuals, following the honest and truthful way in our own lives as in our religious observances. Through Sister Paula, I woke from many of my own cloud-cuckooland about monks and nuns. I previously thought they truly lived 'just' for God and to serve His herd in absolute modesty, following a poverty stricken lifestyle characterized by selflessness. I was dumbfounded to learn that the monastery is not different from any other social-economic or socialistic institute. The Israeli Kibbutz people worked for the kibbutz general needs, and their own needs were supplied by the kibbutz center equally shared with the society so to speak, because they did not earn any money either, yet had all their needs answered. Communism had the same idea when it comes to hard work that one does not get paid for, other than the basic needs the government provides. Nuns do have the benefit of medical insurance, food, a roof over their head and clean clothes (though a uniform but doesn't the army wear uniforms as well and put their life on the line for...?).

So, what is the difference? In my opinion, we are like what Doctor Bruce Lipton so nicely describes in his book, *The Biology of Belief.* Just like cells, our society congregates to work together for a common goal. The main difference I see is this: We have the option to educate ourselves and if we choose, discard old schools that don't suit our present life conditions anymore. We have the ability to change in order to prolong our life—not with medical life support, plugged in, breathing, not living, but rather by creating the proper modifications and adjustments we need for the here and now. (The body's cells do the same by adjusting, evolving, and even mutating when needed.)

Tradition is great until it becomes a dead end street. Joseph Campbell, the great scholar on human mythologies said, "I think our search is somewhat encumbered by our concept of God. God as a final term is a personality in our tradition, so that breaking past that 'personality' into the transpersonal, whether within one's self or in conceiving of the form beyond forms—although one can't even say form—is blocked by our orthodox training. This is so drummed into us, that the word 'God' refers to a personality. Now, there have been very important mystics who have broke past that.

For instance, there is Meister Eckhart, whose line I like to quote: 'The ultimate leave-taking is the leaving of God for God.' Therefore, I don't suggest we toss out our religious beliefs, I would just like to see people assuming some responsibility for their lives and their interpretation of their own beliefs, rather than leaving it all to the God out there. The pharmaceutical industry threatens with viruses, bacteria, and incurable diseases. The religious fanatics prey on our fear of punishment and hell, and the governments threatens with heavy fines if we don't... fill out the blanks. All of that is done in order to disable and disempower us of control over our own life. God, doctors, politicians, or even viruses and bacteria—these are the 'threats' the pharmaceutical companies, the food industry, the churches and religious fanatics use to scare us: On fear to understand and take control over our own lives, health, economy, budget, nutrition, and research. Fear and panic spread like wildfire when our ears hear only the warnings and horrors about the 'Hell' awaiting all those who don't follow God... or medical instructions, failing to take supplements, and heeding the danger of the life-enabling sun.

Sister Paula was a simple woman who just followed. We all have some of Sister Paula in us when we follow. Regardless what and whom, but we do. Sister Paula was struck in disbelief by the misconduct of her bishop and even the Pope's resignation, yet she held fast to her strong beliefs through forgiveness and compassion for the corrupt servants of God of her religious sect. She continued to live, blindly following and believing in everything the church did and ordered until she was forced to change, rebelling against the conservative, mainstream, traditional medicine and convent orders, in order to save her own life. Here she suddenly had to ask herself questions she never would have asked before. If she was such a good nun, why was she being punished? And just like Sister Paula, we don't always have the time to make our own food, rest, deal with our true feelings or the time to be free of media influence and just be in our own selves... until we choose to live otherwise, or like Sister Paula, are forced to.

Sister Paula searched for the magic medicine hoping it would allow her to continue her selfless and destructive lifestyle and still be 'OK' in regards to her congregation and Jesus. But soon she learned that this medicine does not exist. This is exactly why the pharmaceutical companies do so well——because they address precisely this part in us. We would like to be able to close our eyes and without making any changes, expecting a miraculous change will happen. We want to be able to continue striding the same path, which eventually leads us to a point in which no doctor can save us but ourselves, provided we change our route.

The 'do it for us' mentality has taken over since the medicine industry took the driver's seat, and since medicine men and women as well as witches knew all the herbs and poisonous medicinal properties. Yet, now that approach had taken a very lethal turn, since the pharmaceutical companies learned to take complete control, convincing us that we have none. Take for example the 68-year-old man who said to me when his doctor said to him, "Sorry, the hormonal treatments don't seem to work anymore for you and the cancer cells are metastasizing in your prostate." This is what he said to me, "My life is in your hands. I trust you that you will save me." Yet, he would not do his part like drink water, stop smoking or modify his nutrition as I recommended. Cancer is not an evil entity that is out there to get us. Society's structure and our imprisonment in those unnatural social rules, the medical 'quick fix' illusionary false promises, the comforting and emotional numbing industrial food, and fast-paced lifestyles are the bad guys.

We cannot let someone else take care of us or say our own health is all in His hands. We need to grab and hold on to our life's steering wheel to take us where we like to go—good steady and reliable healthy life. Chose our right and wrongs in an educated way and follow that new path. We can make health happen but we have to *choose* the way to our good health and adjust to the necessary changes. We need to change because when we walk the same path, we wind up at the same destination.

In this book I ask you to truly look at yourself and separate the chaff from the stalk. Learn what you should keep from your upbringing and what needs to be changed. Let go or modify that which has been compromising your good health. Think about your religious upbringing, and its unnatural life values. Instead of love and joy we often learn to hate and cherish death and war in the name of God. Look at your outlook about family and work. Why is it so vital to be rich rather than earn money for a comfortable balanced lifestyle? Or like Sister Paula we can chose the semi-poor lifestyle in a very extreme way of self-denial out of fear to run her life by herself. She made her decision at times of war, yet had many years to change that fear based decision in the light of her abundant life conditions and peace. Think about the paths you chose regarding your health, if any.

And please, if at some points you feel I am disrespecting the Catholic Church or any other belief system, please don't meet these sections with anger, but see them as constructive criticism. With an open mind you may find that my point is by no means disrespectful, but rather an examination of what we have been led to believe and how our belief systems can both help and or hurt us. After all, the only guaranteed thing in life is change, and we cannot exclude ourselves from that same rule of nature and have to flow with the changes in life always.

My experience with Sister Paula was for me more instructive than many other experiences I had as a healer with other people who were not devoted and committed to God like a Catholic nun. Sister Paula reflects that extreme part of our society which is deeply entangled in their vows, fears and beliefs because she had lived a life for over fifty years that literally came at the price of her own health and life.

Because everyone has endless access to the vast information through the Internet, we are given an additional challenge to discriminate between the information that is useful and that which is there for dishonest and corrupt purposes. For example, here in the US, we are proud to be the most successful democratic entity in history, yet we are forced by the government to have medical care of the government's choice rather than ours. If we choose the natural health and refuse conventional medicine, which I would never address as medicine to begin with, we are forced to hide from authorities in order to avoid being prosecuted for all the many offenses in their book. We are forced to vaccinate our children in spite of the ten-fold danger we expose our children to, we are 'openly' lied to by the law by paid research and through disregard the obvious autism epidemic and children's old people illnesses. Children's hospitals expand like mushrooms after the rain, and more children are in graveyards today than at any point in the middle ages. We are forced to submit them to medical provider who sees their service as revenue commodity only. And for what purpose? Are they concerned about our health or just a lobbyist's paycheck? Our rights over our own health have been exploited—the sick in our country are wronged every day—and our health is ruled by a government that caters to the pharmaceutical companies owners via the FDA, which in turn is ruled and owned by the pharmaceutical industry—a filthy rich, multibillion dollar enterprise with leaders who care nothing about values, life and integrity, honesty, compassion, health, democracy, future of our nation. Their neglect is obvious as we hit the global record high numbers of obese citizens, the highest number of obesity-related illnesses, autism, cancer and cholesterol, diabetes and high blood pressure sick children, and where are the cancer research results? Every third person dies of cancer, heart disease, or obesity related illness. But we falsely believe we live in a democratic country with freedom of speech, freedom of beliefs, freedom of taking charge over our life, but at what cost?

People, it is time to wake up and think again, doubt, rebel, resist and reclaim our freedom and rights over our life and body, health, and the life of our children. Even Sister Paula realized the injustice, imprisonment, and corruption by the government and medical industry at work, her health as well as in her own higher institute, the Catholic Church in which she believed, but found no power to change.

If we like to believe in God, any God, we are completely free to believe so, but we must also assume responsibility based on our vast knowledge for our own life. You may believe in God without walking in ignorance, the same as our belief in mainstream medicine—we may follow the doctor, but we must not do it ignorantly. We must take the time to listen to our own selves and explore the other ways of living, healing and being.

Attend to your own being and while you are at the wheel rushing to school, work, home, the doctor's office or anywhere you go—turn off your radio, phone or any media you are listening to, and just be in silence for a while. Take the time to listen to yourself.

We have learned how much poison the food industry has smuggled into our food supply in order to reduce their costs and meet a demand that we have blindly created. We want more hamburgers, microwave dinners, easier packaged snacks for our kids—but at what cost? All this rushing around has led us to a life of dining on 'pretend' food. Take a look at the labels next time you buy something to eat… if you don't know what words are on the label of ingredients, then it's safe to say you are not eating what you thought you were buying. Just like the pharmaceutical industry, the food industry as a whole has learned how to cover up all those cheap toxic ingredients. Don't let them play on your "I have no time to prepare my food" melody; rather, change your song. Take responsibility—treasure life. Our doctors today are focused on revenue—including the pure and truthful doctors that are pawns in the bigger scheme. Mainstream medicine is about revenue and not about our life.

My hopes are that through these letters you will ask: What do I believe in, what is driving me to choose my path? Do I blindly follow and believe or do I think and actively pursue my choices? Where is the truth? Do I really need all the medicines I have been taking or could I just change my diet and be more active? Why do I stress over making it to church on Sunday when the rest of my week is spent in the office? How much do I do because it's what I was taught to do? And how much am I doing because I made the choice?

Please approach this book not as a health book or a cancer-healing book, but rather as food for thought for each and every one of us. This book has been written in a new era and new beginnings as the planets Pluto, Neptune, and Uranus moved from the signs they had been for 14 and 20 years.

That means that there must be a revolution of new thinking in every aspect of life, new paths, young, fresh and rebelling attitudes, and understanding of social needs that will all come to surface. It also indicates the clean up of authorities corruption and tyranny. No rock will stay unturned and no lies will prevail. The revolution will be of global magnitude and will go through all and touch all. Change is inevitable as the whole universe is undergoing major transformation. If we don't take our life destiny in our hands and make the necessary changes, changes will do it for us. It is vital for us all to be courageous and initiate any possible change in our life—let go of the out-grown, old, useless cluttering parts in our life and open up and acknowledge our new and true needs, desires, thoughts, realizations, experience and let's go with the flow.

Respectfully,

Yael

Introduction

This story is of a dear friend of mine, Sister Paula. In August of 2007 She was diagnosed with breast cancer and struggled with pressure from her convent to use the mainstream medicine means of cancer treatments although she felt a natural and homeopathic path to healing was best for her. And since a nun should never rebel against the traditional orders and requirements, Sister Paula was very confused and at a loss as to which path she should choose for her alarming health crisis. The cancer diagnosis put her in an entirely new situation. For the first time in her life she had to assume responsibility for herself and her own life and make her own choices about things that at times clashed with her beliefs. She debated whether to use the traditional cancer therapy such as chemotherapy, surgery and radiations, putting her health entirely in the doctor's hands, or choosing, against her convent's approach, to receive cancer therapy the alternative, natural way, which puts her in control.

Sister Paula chose the natural way to health until she reached her goal and at the end of the year of 2007 received a clean bill of health. She continued to live amongst her community of Catholic sisters and never really stopped working with the disabled and challenged adults until her last day. Close to her last days she was struck again by illness and didn't recover from it. Unfortunately, we lost contact from the time she recovered from her breast cancer and was back to her hard working lifestyle in her convent.

I invite you my dear reader to join Sister Paula and I on her interesting, adventurous journey she chose against all rules and orders. I tried not to change her original mail or my own, which both may reflect an accent from our native languages and styles, her Italian and my Hebrew.

When Sister Paula first came to see me prior to her cancer diagnosis, she struggled with severe knee pain and could not find any answer or any medication that helped her. I was very happy to be chosen by a Catholic nun. Being a Jewish born woman, I pictured the nuns as

2

mystical and selfless, knowledgeable, compassionate, and devoted servants to all creation. When Sister Paula arrived for our first meeting, my first impression of her was of the white uniform, her hair tucked neatly under her head covering and a big cross hanging on her chest—she looked sacred and holy, just like a saint to me.

The more skeptical side of me arose, however, when I watched this ancient orthodox, God-serving elderly woman step out of a luxurious, brand new Japanese car. I thought the Catholic Church taught depravity, simplicity and meekness, so I wondered, *Is this what you mean when you say simple living, non-materialistic, owning just the most basic necessities? Does this represent the humble, modest, and poor, a symbol of gratefulness for the little we truly need—not holding on to any possession or personal comfort since the poor people need all we can give?* For the shiny glittery snazzy expensive car did not seem to represent that role model for simplicity and modesty. Yet, when I imagined the luxurious Vatican, I could not see all those alleged values materialized there either.

Sister Paula got my name from a chiropractor that tried to help her for a year or may be even longer with her knee. He and I met when assuming I just needed a neck adjustment after a car accident. He looked at me and said, "I worked in a biological research lab for a few years prior to my present career. I know what you have is not a dislocated neck; it is the West Nile virus." Yep, it took me another little struggle to overcome this one too, but this is how my story with Sister Paula was seeded.

Sister Paula was overweight as she told me about her knees, and about her hard work at the center for disabled adults. Apparently to ease all the hardship, sweets, coffee and cake, a lot of pasta and other baked goods (especially since she was of Italian descent and was living in an Italian convent) were her weaknesses. Our conversations were very easy and my awe of a Catholic nun in my office melted away pretty soon opening a path for person-to-person chat between us.

Sister Paula was very shy and obedient and promised to do her best to closely follow my recommendations to contribute to her own health. Needless to say how hard it was on both of us to find a common ground and materialize those changes – you will see those reasons in the following email exchange. Eventually, Sister Paula reached her goal: A clean bill of health, but to my dismay, resumed her old traditional habits and therefore did not hold onto her good health for much longer.

Soon she stopped considering her own needs, sacrificing her sleep, her nutrition and even resuming her deep anger with the center's management, which were her biggest problems bringing her to that poor health in the first place. I only know that once she had her clean bill of health, she got very upset when I reminded her not to neglect herself again, and then she disconnected.

Sister Paula expressed her gratefulness for my suggestion to publish our email exchange as she realized how helpful they might be for others who have been diagnosed with breast cancer.

I am grateful for her kind permission to publish our very intimate and candid emails.

Chapter 1: The Journey Begins

These next few email exchanges we find the first cracks in the walls of believers like Sister Paula, as she suddenly faces adversity in everything she stood for and faithfully followed, as meeting me thanks to her knee pain reflected to her a very different view of life she found impossible to accept. Every one of us wakes up at a certain point in life to see how life demands changes in order to continue. For some of us it is nature's transition and in those of us, like Sister Paula it is about life and death.

July 3, 2007

Dear Dr. Yael,

This new month of July 2007 is my 73rd birthday and a big number, which gives me one more powerful reason to assess my life and the direction in which I am striding. To explain my life as a nun is a little difficult for my poor expression assets. In our last meeting I sensed how different your life is compared to mine, in a way that I never realized before. Your suggestions and guidance, however, are precious to me. I realize how fortunate I am (and they are many) as to know you as one of the greatest gifts from God in my life. The richness of the Word of God that every day is given to me in abundance is another gift on which I am going to concentrate more, and let the Word of the Lord, to whom I committed my whole life, be my strength. My health is good; my knees do not hurt as much thanks to your help, and my diet? Well, I have to work at it more since it requires me to 'swim' against our cultural trend. (I am Italian, as you know, and living among the Italians makes dieting very difficult.) I will be away from home the next two weeks, for a brief vacation and traveling which does not help my nutrition regime.

I keep you in my prayers every day and also think about your book, *Giggling Dr. Green*, for the revolution it will bring, as well as your courage to write it!

Love and Blessings—

Sister Paula

July 17, 2007

Dear Dr. Yael,

On Sunday I returned from my retreat/vacation/break and was very happy to find your so vibrant and friendly e-mail. During these past days I often thought about you, especially in prayer, and wish to share with you my wonderful experience in my search for God. Your idea of writing a book about a nun's life is wonderful, but we should have the opportunity to talk more. My life (that you correctly perceive as submissive to tradition) is also filled with a great freedom in my sanctification to God and my vows to poverty, chastity and obedience. This is the quintessence of our religious life.

The danger of this freedom of the spirit that should move the person constantly upwards, is in becoming a routine, as even the most sacred things that I come in contact with, like the Sacred Scripture or the Sacraments, do not bring me closer to God. Sometimes I feel like I'm living in a continuous struggle against mediocrity,

9

superficiality and anger. But I know that God loves me and called me to a life of holiness, and in spite of all those human weaknesses and obstacles, He is faithful to His promises.

I do not know how close I am to God; I only trust His mercy.

Are you going to have a signing ceremony when your book published? I would really like to be there. I have to go now—Thank you for all your kindness

Love,

Sister Paula

July 21, 2007

Dear Sister,

Thank you for your e-mail. It feels good to have this wonderful spiritual connection with you. I realize that you don't have a lot of free time to spend with me but when you do it feels blessed, good and mighty. I will definitely tell you if and when I will have any event coming up for my book, *Giggling Dr. Green.* The editor is writing to me about how powerful this book is and how she felt it was sent to her from God, how she is honored to edit it. I am so grateful to be blessed by, and carry the message of, truth, honesty and integrity to the children through my book.

I love you and thank you for being in my life—
Yael
July 22, 2007

Dear Dr. Yael,

11

It is true, I do not have much time to spend on the computer, but I do like to write to you and to receive your letters. I would like to begin this e-mail with the phrase you used in your closing, "I love you and thank you for being in my life."

Today, Sunday, is the day of the Lord. I spent half of my day in Church in prayers, songs, listening, meditating the Word of God and participating in the sacred rituals. It is a beautiful opportunity in my life that completes my weekly activities. I am not going to do great things, everything in my life is simple, but I believe that all we do is great if it is done with love. Since I answered the call to follow Jesus Christ, I know that if I am faithful to Him and His teachings, everything I do has the redemptive power of His death and Resurrection. I do not know if you ever had the opportunity to read the Gospel, because it is amazing how much I find in your moral and religious values that are the very spirit of the Gospel.

Thank you again for being in my life.

These days, the Catholic Church is going through a period of darkness, locally, nationally and internationally. But it is still Holy, Universal and Apostolic. It is composed of humans and as we all know, we make mistakes and sin, but the foundation of the Church is Jesus and He is God. I thank God every day for belonging to the Catholic Church and this year, in 2007, I celebrate fifty years of religious life.

I received a message last week about my older sister in Italy, that she is seriously ill and that the whole family worries about her. She is eighty years old. I placed her in God's hands, to give her strength and peace to follow His will, whatever it will be. Please remember her in your prayers. There is a great spiritual writer that summarizes all our life struggles in a simple sentence:

"At the end of life we will be judged only by our love." (John of the Cross)

With love and prayers,
Sister Paula

July 23, 2007

Dear Sister Paula,

Thank you for your soul soothing words that never regard money, politics or business issues, but faith and values, prayers and love. All are values the world should follow instead of the greed, fear, political affairs, power struggles, ego and inequitable businesses, which are very unethical standards and evidently are very contagious even for the churches, synagogues and mosques as we both see. It is correct, as you say that Catholicism is not the people but the idea of God. Like Jehovah are not the Jewish people but the understanding of God's values, and the same goes for Allah and its followers. Consequently, it is so important to keep in mind those who slip simply could not control their weaknesses, yet still could find God in those same weaknesses if they chose. For that reason God is in us and must be served and cannot be replaced. Given that God is Love and people make mistakes and struggle with

14

their weaknesses and fears, they lose the love in those struggles.

I never read the Gospel, but I have read the Old Testament numerous times and when I talk to you I talk from my heart and my core beliefs. I strongly believe that God is in every one of us and so we *are* God and those who do not follow his guidance simply do not follow their own guidance, which I call consciousness. Those who never open their eyes to see where God really is are poor souls that make their mistakes and are searching for God out there, and they wonder why they don't find him or her. I believe that when Jesus Christ died he had such a mighty soul, enough to spread his message and values among all of humanity. So no one needs to look for him out there, but rather within one's self. By looking into ourselves we find love, kindness, forgiveness, tolerance, gratefulness, compassion, mercy, appreciation and remorse. And as we do find all of those, we know we found God. And once we found God we have no fear anymore and no revulsion, resentment, covetousness, rage; those godless feelings

15

simply dissolve and disappear… like you wrote about your sister, and your wishes to allow God do what is best for her body and soul, her love and compassion. Finding God is accepting life as we go along, learning and seeing the wisdom in everything that comes our way on this journey. I think this is the way to find God, joy and acceptance in whatever life has to offer us.

When Moses looked down Mount Sinai he saw his people dance around the golden calf and he thus shattered the Ten Commandments (according to the Bible). He realized that his people were not ready yet to find God on the intellectual and spiritual plane. He became their spiritual mentor to guide them in learning about the intangible God, unlike the Egyptian statues and goddesses they knew. Moses lead his people through the Sinai Desert for forty years knowing it would take a whole generation, or even longer, before these men and women would be ready for the Ten Commandment – the rules of higher social values and the way of finding God. To evolve means to accept and understand ethics and ways of life as dictated by the Bible. Instead of an unrestrained desire, fury, hatred, distrust and retribution based society, they had to learn and assimilate higher spiritual standards as an alternative.

Now, all religions are at the same evolutionary intersection. Christianity, the Catholic Church, Judaism and Islam must reestablish and redefine the true divine ideals, return to genuineness and be keen on wasted actions of voracity and dishonesty, give up the self serving substance benefits; they must not use God's name in vain to feed their animalistic desires and rather resume trustworthy deeds. They must discontinue the molestation of young children and end the embezzlements and other acts of greed and selfishness so that the fundamental morals and rules of our evolved society can prevail. It is for the whole world to know that no matter (calf equals dollar signs) or person, even when wearing a royal cloak, can replace our human society values, as we are – God.

Everything else is nothing more than valueless, ego driven, dishonest and corrupted low lives, leeching on society in their faulty services. God is mighty and has many

17

names; nevertheless, the only way to find him is in kindness, love, and service to his creation, truth, nature, smiles and compassion. Not through any other kind of material means and hateful and malicious destructive conduct. God exists in every sunray, in a caring touch of men, or a flower and animal to help. I find God in each drop of water enabling my existence and stilling my thirst, in the blossoms before bearing fruit to ease my hunger. This is how I feel and find the divine and pay my thanks each day and every moment. I believe that once we all discover these enlivening secrets there will be no war, no drugs, no hunger, no sadness and no greed or crime. People will lose interest in saturation of anything like possession, too much food, or sex; in the clutter they need ever bigger closets and trash cans, as they find no comfort or satisfaction in the excess any more. They may find no need for false pride and this change will evoke the relaxing and healing properties in the simple natural life: food, pure water and in the smile of a child or friend.

Dear Sister, thank you for being here to invite my thoughts. And since thoughts become things, may they travel around the universe, touch many more good souls like you and enter more hearts in order to bring peace and love.

Please write again for your words are meaningful to me and to the whole world. Let's keep our good work and prayers.

Love,

Yael

July 29, 2007

Dear Dr. Yael,

First let me thank you for your beautiful long letter. I really enjoyed reading it and even printed it so that I can return to it in my quiet moments. Sharing your great faith and core beliefs is challenging and reassuring as you speak about the only true meaning of our lives. What can I share with you? I am not a writer but I will put in words how wonderful it is to live a life consecrated to God only, as the ultimate purpose. Thus it does not insinuate being isolated from the surrounding world and its difficulties. I feel it as part of humanity's sinful daily struggle to be faithful. But I know how God is close to me and is faithful to His promises. By beginning each day praising the Lord, to witness His love and His presence through my very simple activities, to teach my students and my co-workers, the children and people in my church, His love and His truth, and to end each day by thanking the Lord for all that happened during that day, is a privilege that makes me say

20

like the words of the Psalm: "What shall I render unto God for all His mercy."

Last Friday was July 20th and by the Church's calendar, on this day we remember two great figures of the Old Testament: Joachim and Anna, the parents of Mary, Jesus' mother. In my prayer I clearly remembered the 20th of July fifty years ago when I was on the Alps, Italy's mountains. I stood at the top viewing the most beautiful scenery one can imagine and on that day I clearly and powerfully experienced that calling of Jesus to follow Him. Since that day I went through a lot of struggles and difficulties on the road following Jesus, but with His Love and the life He has sacrificed for me, every day, the entire way I traveled through the sacred ceremonials and the Word, I am still holding onto Him. He is the rock of my salvation and the only way I believe in deliverance for humankind. I feel very close to you when you talk about finding God in a smile, in the beauty of a flower, in the refreshing gift of water and the air. Our earth is the most beautiful gift God has given us, and now we have to learn to preserve and protect it from destruction, greed and ignorance.

I am concluding with an excerpt from the Gospel by Matthew to illustrate how close you are to the spirit of the Gospel in your beliefs: "Jesus said: Look at the birds in the sky. They do not sow or reap; they gather nothing into barns; yet your heavenly Father feeds them. Are not you more important than they? Learn your lessons from the way the flowers of the field grow. They do not work; they do not spin. Yet I assure you, not even Solomon in all his splendor was arrayed like one of these. If God can clothe in such splendor the grass of the field, which blooms today and is thrown in the fire tomorrow, will He not provide much more for you? Stop worrying like the none believers, your heavenly Father knows all your needs." (Matthew 7:26-31)

I thank you for your friendship and for helping me to re-examine my life by revealing myself to you.

Love and prayers,

Sister Paula

July 30, 2007

Dear Sister,

Here you can see how successfully and ingenuously you have written to me despite your doubts. Though I have never read the Gospel it struck me how limitless and boundless energy actually is in time and space, something that even religions cannot detain as religions are created by men rather than part of the universe or nature. For all that is happening, is here and now. God and divinity – nature is present, never aging and never leaving. Only we the people think the world today does not belong to yesterday and tomorrow. (Just like mainstream medicine lets us believe that the leg is not connected to the eye and that cancer is a 'chemotherapy and radiation' deficiency.) Only we humans can imagine that the earth belongs to us to deplete and abuse instead of trusting that the earth actually lands us a little time and space to stay here for a while and enjoy all the gifts we are presented with before continuing on our soul's journey. God – Universe – Divinity – Nature – our

23

beliefs... never ends and never begun. Nobody can see, smell or touch them and they are eternal. Only those who can see the divinity in the flowers and the birds, the sea and the clouds, can see the divine, nature's order, supervision and grace.

Think: Have you ever tried to count the water drops you have been drinking? Or the precious water drops running down your body while standing under your daily shower? All those are nature's divinity, yet we never stop for a moment and count them because we take them for granted as if they were meant to be there for us. I believe that the universe is touching us with its elixir of life. I know that without energy, this universal wisdom, there is no life. Therefore, water, a flower, a precious little baby, every tree and lizard and butterfly, all the love and hope- mean life. Without those, no life can exist. When I say 'God' I mean waking up in the morning and saying, "I am," meaning "nature's divine energy of the universe." There is no difference between thousands of years ago and now. Then people needed compassionate and merciful leaders to guide them to wisdom and love and help them separate from fear, greed, and anger, jealousy and evil. And today people are not different.

Thank you for sharing your memories with me of the time you were still a young girl in Italy. Speaking of Italy, how is your biological sister? Please, write again when you have time and let me know if I can be any help to you.

(By the way, though Jesus said not to worry God is providing everything, when Adam and Eve were pushed out of the Garden of Eden God said to Adam,

"In the sweat of thy face

shalt thou eat bread, till

thou return unto the ground")

Love,

Yael

August 2, 2007

My Dear Dr. Yael,

Thank you for your last reply that I enjoyed so much. I am always amazed and inspired by your deep connection to God through nature and by the simplicity of your approach, which identifies you so close with the spirit of the Gospel. Jesus said, "If you do not become like little children, you cannot enter the kingdom of God." Many people have to struggle all their life to acquire this spirit of total trust in God, like a child that rests secure in his mother's arms, and here you are in your expressions revealing this great virtue strong and clear. Another surprise in your letter was when you mentioned the Holy Spirit. As a Catholic nun I believe in the Holy Spirit, which is very important in my life as the source and giver of life, the counselor, the advocate, the fire of Love, and more... Going back to the Gospel, after Jesus rose from death and before ascending into heaven, He promised to send the Holy Spirit to guide and strengthen His disciples in their

26

mission (John 14:18-26). And the Holy Spirit came on the day of Pentecost, and His presence was felt as a strong wind and as flames of fire. That was the beginning of the Church and since then the Holy Spirit comes to each believer through the rituals, beginning with Baptism. As you said, the Holy Spirit is always present among us and His spiritual gifts that help us to live the message of Jesus were already listed in the book of the Prophet Isaiah. From the Old to the New Testament, the Spirit of God makes us really one people without a division of categories; all are called to be part of His life.

Thank you for remembering my sister; she is doing better, recuperating slowly and probably in need of surgery for her liver in the near future. As for myself, I am doing very well; my knees do not hurt any more (thank you). I took the homeopathic drops you gave me a few times, I concentrate more on the spiritual values, renewed my faith and trust in God so that the disappointing and frustrating situations in my professional life do not upset me so much any more. I must admit that I have to be more consistent in my diet. Sometimes I forget, sometimes I am too hungry and I always eat too fast and too much. That is my weakness and I have to better. Can you help me with that? I must go now; I would like to talk to you forever but let the Spirit do that for us.

Love and blessing,

Sister Paula

Reflections

After the exchange of love emails I start to tap into the natural healing kingdom, which created even a bigger conflict in Sister Paula as she started to get seriously ill.

The biggest dilemma she faced was - the clash between her decades old beliefs and her present reality. And where is the lord? Can God be nature? Or can nature be god?

Sister Paula feared her soul freedom because that would, in her eyes, distance her from the total belief and submission to Jesus. She could not fathom herself think for herself, and make her own choices for her health. Sister Paula's way of life was based completely and absolutely on servicing god. Though she understood how nature is she and she was part of nature, it didn't really manifested in her actuality. This distance from her natural needs and rights, alienated her emotional as well as physical needs, desires, and health to a total denial. We cannot live outside our being and in complete declination to ourselves. We never, in any stage of our life "outgrow" our little child in us. This

29

part in our being will always stay with us, and if we deny it and never attend to it, we will get sick. This is the problem with the mainstream medicine, and the big difference between my approach and theirs. The illness will appear only when we let it. Only when we don't listen and cater to our needs, whether they are emotional and/or physical needs. And thus, when a sick individual seeks my help, I will never treat the symptoms before I get to the reason for his or her illness.

One of the best examples was a 40 years old man who came to me in excruciating pains in his hands feet and spine. He told me about the horrible side effects he suffered from the pain killer medications, and bagged for help. He showed me how swollen his hands and fingers were and how he couldn't even hold his toothbrush. As we talked about how and when those intolerable pain and swelling started, I heard his anger at his sister and her spouse who were in the same business with him. I never gave him a homeopathic remedy for his joints and swelling, but for his anger. This anger was denied and tucked in. His body developed the exact same hormones like in war or big danger. However, he never took the time to relax and to do any physical activity, which would help him break down those acidic secretions. Those latter accumulated in his joints and caused that violent inflammation. A few months past before I saw him again, but this time he was smiling and happy. He told me how he started to workout every day, he took the remedy I gave him and learned to balance between work and fun time and relaxation as well.

His joints were now completely free, his muscles nicely sculptured and he enjoyed good health.

He also revealed to me the major changes in his diet he made, and learned to speak out if matters were disagreeable. Sister Paula got so used to her submission and acceptance that she just followed, but never decided for herself any matter in her life. Her frustrations seemed to her as sinful, and so she numbed her feelings by binging on unhealthy food. It served her wrong on both ends, denial caused her inner toxicity, and the unhealthy food cased her over weight and constant inflammation. This is what happens to us all if we deny our little child the basic vital needs. In life we need a healthy balance of, nutrition, time to relax and play, time to rest and sleep, share and give to others, yet not to forget our own needs. If we have no one to share our feelings, we must admit them to ourselves and address them in a constructive way.

Even the so basic sexual desires were denied, and those are a vital life saving hormonal needs every living creature has. To deny them the way sister Paula has for her entire life, of course changes her hormonal equilibrium and result in illness. I don't suggest that we can disregard our daily duties and responsibilities. I also don't suggest that there are times in life in which we have to step up to adversity and bite through it. What I do suggest is, watch the little children, though they have their difficulties and problems (we may sometimes even underestimate) they soon retrieve into their dollhouse, or basketball or painting and dive into their kingdom of relaxation, creativity and happy imagination. We should take them as our most important mentor in regards to relaxation and cater to our inner child in order to stay healthy and balanced. If you can play silly after work, or go play basketball, or knit, or paint, you will save the money for a psychiatrist, and will never suffer illness, depression or stress related illnesses. I paint, dance, sing, knit, practice qigong and tai chi, go for walks, play silly with my grandchildren, and meditate outdoors.

I never had to take a blood pressure or cholesterol medication. Thus, I also never binge on toxic food to numb my emotions. I prefer to write, and move, talk and cry, if necessary.

I like you to adapt something constructive and enjoyable to release stress and keep your inner child's voice heard.

Please understand that though from the outside Sister Paula and alike seem to live the perfect life, they do not. They live in total deafness to their natural vital needs, and in my humble opinion, serving god doesn't mean killing the creatures he created in his own image.

Chapter 2: Overcoming Doubt

When we blindly follow our religious guides and fail to see the universal connections between all. Sister Paula biggest challenge is to take a step away from her lifelong beliefs and peek into the world from a different angle.

Sister Paula learns that we must see, hear and discover and at times even suffer or experience joy without any doubt because we know that there must be a higher purpose for everything, a bigger plan than we possibly know or can view from our tiny spot on the earth, thus part of the entire universe.

Only if Sister Paula will conquer her fear and step out of her little box will she be able to heal.

In this chapter Sister Paula listens, or reads about the different aspects and philosophies yet dares not to make the vital changes to save her life.

Undoubtedly we all have those conflicts and some of us pay the heavy price of fear of change, with our precious life.

August 5, 2007

Dear Sister,

You probably know that according to the Old Testament, when the Israelites had to leave Egypt, the Holy Spirit was the fire pillar that ran before the expedition to guide, protect and inspire the people through the desert. So, why would I not mention the Holy Spirit? It is not just the Catholic privilege or invention. It is part of the Jewish tradition and beliefs as well.

Your e-mail brings me back to a session I had with a friend of mine who is a guided imaginary practitioner, or also called visualization therapist. Visualization therapy helps us to reprogram the brain by letting go of old negative memories and emotions and replacing them with a positive approach to life challenges. At one of those sessions she guided me into a deep self-hypnotic state in which I regressed into one of my past lives. This was my internal vision:

I was in a park in front of a very old big building. It could have been the 17th century, or 18th, (I had no calendar with me) and it was a very gloomy, very cold and strange place. I saw nuns in gray garments with very great head coverings resembling in my imagination, wings on both sides of their head. In the center stood a big birch tree surrounded by a spiked iron fence and the nuns hurried on their bicycles to the big building. It was very chilly and hazy as the sun came down and it felt as if nobody knew one another, as if everything was outlandish. A few older couples were holding onto each other's arms in a slow pace, wearing their monocles and warm jackets, and the ladies in their long dresses and tight, somewhat elegant, and appropriate hats on, were striding beside the men. Everyone was serious, the colors were gray and the pace was very slow, weird and saturnine.

I saw myself lying on a heavy wooden framed bed in a minimally furnished room, nothing but very simple, old wooden furniture. Only the necessities were there, like a straight back, rustic oak chair, a clear-cut small nightstand for a candle at my bedside, and everything was built of thick logs, unembellished and crude. That huge empty room was constructed of wood and was not pleasing to the eye or the imagination. There was no decoration, no pictures or ornament. Large dark beams were running along the ceiling for support, complementing the timber floor. The only decoration was a cross hanging on the wall over my head with Jesus made of wood on the bare wall. I was lying on an extremely hard and thin mattress. Everything was incredibly quiet along with a holy and sacred mood. I was lying there awaiting my death.

A beautiful young nun was sitting quietly at my side holding my hand and her eyes were filled with love as she was watching me with her serious young look, in spite of her eyes filled with tears she seemed peaceful and content. I could feel by the way she was holding my hand, and saw it in her eyes, that she was waiting for a sign from me asking for anything she could go and bring me. I recognized her, for she is my grand daughter of today in this life. Omrie lives in Israel. In that incarnation I was a nun and was dying of old age without any fear or anguish but with acceptance and thanks. I sensed the warmth and love pour into me from her youthful loving sensitive hands as she thanked me for being her mentor and older sister for all those years. You were around in that covenant too and together we worshiped and served.

Now, whenever we mention the Holy Spirit it takes me back to my previous life when my soul was still learning, as my visits here on planet earth is my soul journey, evolution and mission. This is how I experience life and this is my conviction for as long as I can recall. Now, referring to Jesus' words, it carries me back in time and feels so real, although it is just my imagination. Who knows? Could it be that my soul was there? This experience is elating and magic and reading your quotes on top of it also demonstrates to me the resemblance to my words. It is awesome.

The very controversial book, at least for the Catholics and Christians, *The Da Vinci Code*, reminded me of the same place as in my past life experience, with a pretty vivid sensation of the higher spirit and divinity. Do I sound slightly insane? However, all prophets were thought to be insane, so I am in good company. The prophets' missions and speeches to their people were visions and thoughts and they expressed their enlightenments and revelations, nevertheless, people were oblivious. Though I don't consider myself a prophet or a leader I do encounter people's comments suggesting that I am "living on a different planet" when they are listening to me. My attitude and ways of thinking enable me to rise above the mundane 'soul polluting' current circumstances, as the TV commercials or meaningless programs of gossip play in the background. In this way I can unchain myself from those and take a view of life and the world from an 'astronaut point of view.' It gives me a clean mind that allows me to help people in uncommon and different ways other than the mainstream medicine, or even different than many other alternative medicine practitioners. Health practitioners who are restricted and limited to the schools requirements and instructors' opinions continue as they were trained to think and are apprehensive to 'jump out of the box' leaving no room for their healer's intuition. After all, the art of healing depends upon the healer's knowledge and intuition, his or her ability to listen and understand the person by reading his body language and to attend to his deepest fears, his disappointments and the difficulties he is facing. A true skillful healer will help his patient restore joy in life, the true gift of health.

I am convinced that respecting our inner child is essential in our search for happiness and substantial well-being, and allows us to celebrate the universe's endless abundance. Only if we value nature and know that this is who we are and, as we maintain our humble and grateful attitude, keep honoring and accepting the paths of life, we will never suffer need, just like the tree-house that makes a child feel as though it is a real home and the most beautiful and best palace in the world. In their nature, kids are completely content and happy with what they have and can create something we adults often miss out.

The main difference between the young ones and us is that they merely create more in their imagination and find comfort, coziness, safety and satisfaction there. Little do we realize how everything we try so desperately to hold on to and fight for is nothing but our own illusions and if we choose, we can imagine even our small and simple home is a palace; our apple and sandwich with a glass of water in the park becomes our feast in a fancy restaurant. It is all in our mind and our perception and our attitude. Only if we could retrieve to the skillful abilities of a young enthusiastic child, could we possibly be truly happy and most of all— would stay healthy.

Love and thankfulness lead to wealth because of the universe's law of attraction: Like attracts like. The universe provides us with the whole lot and only appreciation can conduct us to bliss and ecstasy. Subsequently, we are capable of finding the kindness and generosity of the creation. At this stage we can see how the divine is here in us and for us, and not out there in heaven or on any throne or sanctuary, cross or church. If we struggle and encounter hardship, whether with our surrounding relatives and friends or at work or at home, or even on the road, we know that we—the universe—are learning a little lesson for our soul's evolution rather than being 'punished' by God, because God does not inhibit us from learning. Our experiences direct us so we can see, ascertain and progress, even if not for an obvious visible reason. It may be part of the larger plan and the better and bigger picture, possibly even for our next life, or if you like—the next stage in our soul's evolution. Or for the mission we carry as one of the angels that serve the cosmos and creation. So, we must see, hear and discover and at times even suffer or experience joy without any doubt because we know that there must be a higher purpose for everything, a bigger plan than we possibly know or can view from our tiny spot on the earth, thus part of the entire universe.

With love,

Yael

August 11, 2007

Dear Dr. Yael,

Your last e-mail has really amazed me and I agree that sometimes you sound like a person from another planet. Maybe you had previous different lives as you experienced in the visualization therapy; personally I do not believe it but that is just for myself. I had the opportunity to practice visualization therapy during one of my retreats a few years ago, which helped me to better know myself and see more clearly my limitations and strengths on the other hand. Knowing and sharing my faith and beliefs with you presently is beautiful and I go through a sensation of a mysterious bond with you I cannot explain or understand. But I am living only in the present; I have only this life to spend for God, following the call of Jesus my Savior through the teachings of the Gospel.

The Gospel is the "Word of God." It is part of the Bible and has been recognized as the inspired revelation of God to mankind. The book you mentioned, *The Da Vinci*

Code, I purposely have not read partially because it is fiction. There are many books and movies about Jesus mixing sacred history with fiction and by reading them we must be careful not to take them as the "Inspired Revelation," but only as somebody's opinion or fantasy. I am closing this mail with a quotation from the Gospel in which Jesus said, "Blessed are the pure in spirit for they shall see God." And this verse is like an explanation or a further clarification of Psalm 24 in the Old Testament, "The Lord is the earth and its fullness, who shall climb the mountain of the Lord? Who shall stand in his holy place? The man with clean hands and a pure heart does not desire worthless things and never deceives his neighbor."

May God bless you and fill you with his love and presence always.

With love and prayers—
Sister Paula

August 12, 2007

Dear Sister Paula,

I agree with you about the fiction, however I also believe that God reveals him or herself to us in so many unexpected ways and images. Like in the beauty of every tree and the beauty of a newborn calf, in the power of nature men cannot harness, in the ability to heal and regain power and courage, in so many innumerable ways. I usually don't read science fiction yet still this book grabbed my attention. It gave me a mysterious feeling of how even though I was born Jewish, I can still feel connectedness and love for Jesus. I even felt how human he was and how we all are actually connected and we are all one. We all are light and energy and thrive from love and care. If feelings like these can be reached through a science fiction book in a Jewish person, or any other person in the world that did not grow up Catholic, or in someone that doesn't know much about the Catholic religion, it carries a message that is imperative to every reader. The book is not trying to convert its readers to Christianity or Catholicism, but it successfully conveys the message of oneness. God only knows if this book was written for that purpose or maybe for any different purpose and possibly—a key one. See, if I only open my heart to the universe's guidance, I am able to follow for this is in my eyes what we consider as—coincidence. I trust that just like the red flower has its color and the bluebird is blue for a reason nature assigned it and the geese migrate every winter from Canada and the ocean is harnessed to the shores and boundaries, we human are part of the world of nature just alike. I believe that though we may be able to control that which is happening to us, and since the Universe is we and our love and nature, so in reality (if there is a reality as we understand it) nature or universe or cosmos controls our life. This has always led me to stay open and receptive to whatever comes my way until eventually it dawned on me; it must be the awareness and immersion with the universal wisdom and guidance that explains our intuition, wisdom, and comprehension. And here is a little story:

Four years ago we applied for my husband's permanent residency here in the US.

Many unforeseen errors kept our goal from materializing, like for example; the judge forgot to date one of the documents when signing it, or the attorney misplaced certificates and so on. The attorney's sloppy job aggravated my husband who felt that the attorney's wife's, as well as his negligence (they worked together in their law firm) and their failure to detect the incomplete documents kept us for another year and a half from going back home to visit our family. We were scheduled for another hearing at the immigration office after the attorney, allegedly, thoroughly checked all the documents to assure us there would be no more errors this time. But low and behold the case had to be rescheduled once again for more 'little question marks' the immigration officer had overlooked, which of course meant that we had to patiently wait a few more months for the next hearing.

As our attorney entered the INS waiting room he looked troubled (but not for our sake) and told us about

47

the bad news his wife received that morning. The news about her father's illness and that he was diagnosed with pancreatic, liver and kidney cancer and was sent home to die. This lady was my husband's reason for his frustration and anger since she disregarded her responsibility of her job, which caused our delay. Now her father was on his deathbed and she was of course very sad and devastated. As the attorney talked about his father-in-law's dreadful treatments and hopelessness I suggested a more natural way knowing that it may only give him a better life quality for the time he has left. I also shared with the attorney how at times, when mainstream medicine runs out of resources and can not help anymore, there may still be a lot that nature has to offer, especially since the doctors lack the tools once chemotherapy, surgery and radiation don't work anymore. I thought there were still some things that could benefit him in order to prolong his life, even if for just a few more months or years yet, the father would be free of pain and suffering. The attorney looked at me very skeptically and doubtfully, something he could not or maybe even would not try to hide. I said nothing more.

Later that day his wife (the 'bad' attorney) called me and begged me to come and see her father. She was sobbing throughout his whole session and then said to me: "Is God punishing me for the mistake I made with your husband?"

"Of course not," was my prompt reply. "The way I understand it, God never punishes, but we are scolding ourselves. I am certain that although we don't always understand the universe's bigger plan, the universe harbors no anger and no ill feelings and has no false ego issues like we humans have, and since we are God and we are the universe, it is our own ego and false pride which is our harsh teacher. It rather feels as if the universe kept us here in the US in an elegant way to fulfill the mission to try and save one of us."

It took just a few foot massage and homeopathy treatments, pulse electromagnetic therapy and some nutrition modification, for her father to get out of bed, take

49

longer walks in his neighborhood and feel better. All his vital functions gradually regenerated. It looked as if he got out of harm's way for the time being. Only if we could retrieve to the skillful abilities of a young enthusiastic child, could we possibly be truly happy and most of all—would stay healthy for years. His daughter revealed to me in confidentiality that he had been unfaithful to his wife, her mother. That mistake he made many years earlier created a gap between he and his wife, which kept them from reconciling their marriage. A forty-year-old daughter born out of wedlock kept adding 'salt on their wounded souls' for all those years. The resentment and isolation they endured had left an incurable scar in both who once were a loving happy couple, and along with his infidelity, caused his self sentence to die in suffering.

I always see whatever happens must be for a reason even if we don't see it yet. I don't suggest that it was his illness he had to bare, though it sure served many seemingly unrelated aspects. It seems as if his wife, who was a registered nurse in the oncology department, had the opportunity to learn a different approach to cancer patients and said to me that all she sees are just ends and no hope on every shift she works. Her daughter had learned about her father's infidelity and how, although sinful, he was her father and she loved and forgave him. She also saw how we must "love our neighbor like thyself" and do our very best when we work and serve because we never know when we might need our client and in turn become his or her client. Her father had to learn how self-scolding is a dangerous curse and we should rather converse, apologize and manage our anger with those we had hurt. The skeptical attorney watched how powerful nature is and how we must keep our heart and mind open for the unknown.

My husband learned that nothing happens in vain, even if our path happens to be blocked for a while and we have to await the change. Our relationship would never continue to exist had he not been held from leaving as he would rather controlled by his impulse to get up and leave when things did not go his way. He had to stay six long years and buff his ego horns and learn to handle our partnership in a more mature manner, rather than the childish way before. He learned that his paperwork, like his names and documents, were in such array and turned out they were the true reason for all the confusions and delays he so hated with his passionate impassions. It was an important schooling for him to learn to respect the law and keep his sensitive certificates in a safe place. He lives with me today with kindness, appreciation and contentment, happy the INS blocked his 'escape route.'

The attorney's entire family learned how to view cancer without fear, and instead found they would alternate their lifestyle if they were to be diagnosed. They all had the opportunity to learn cancer prevention methods as well as preventions for other degenerative illnesses of our time. The purpose of this strange INS delay conveyed endless healing opportunities and may even continue to flow in directions we may never know. Yes, it had a very meaningful purpose without any doubt. This lady just nodded and could not stop praising my work, commitment and success with her father for the next few months and said to me, "How will I ever be able to thank you for still having my father? He doesn't suffer and still functions. I know he will not live forever, but he is here and smiles."

Then a year later he passed on and she never exchanged another word with me; she was just furious. Could all that be the reason for the strange chain of events that kept us from leaving the US at that particular time? Only the universe knows.

If Dan Brown wrote his book, *The Da Vinci Code*, he probably, even maybe unknowingly and unaware, was guided to write it. In everything we create, whether it is a good dish, writing a poem or a book, creating a piece of art, we must be inspired in a way to deliver a certain mission or message for the world. Universe is a creator and every creation is part of this energy, and so is creation.

Intuitively I was guided to read this writing and though Jewish born, it taught me love for the Gospel and recognition of Jesus as a healing sole and great teacher. It feels blissful to open my eyes and heart to these new revelations. Whether my discoveries came from a Disney movie or were revealed to me in a children's book or in a science fiction book makes no difference. As you know, by being in touch with the world around us we are able to learn from anyone and everything. I am still a child in the cosmos, which allows me to be open hearted to any marvelous experience and perhaps get one more hint to connect and unite me with the divine, to the history, to the oneness and to the Gospel. It is not about the book's direct message or teachings; it is about its byproduct stimulating the interest in the harmony and our connectedness. I realize that this is another very long email, but important when considering the "mysterious connection with you." You had mentioned that before, and it makes me thankful and respectful.

Regards,
Yael

Reflections

Sister Paula and I had beautiful heartwarming email exchange, and I must admit that it surpassed the typical doctor patient relationship. I was very open and private in my letters to her, and felt towards her more as a close spiritual soulmate, rather than just professional person. The truth is that I could and did feel that since money never changed hands, I could take the liberty and treat her and our relationship with as much love as I felt.

Sister Paula was my 'secret little friend' who I could join into her sanctuary and absorb that purity of soul and her close connection to the holiness I always dreamed about. As I described already, churches always gave me that inner feeling of closeness to the higher mighty creator, whoever it might be. I am aware of my childish needs; I would be happy to ride in Cinderella's pumpkin courage or hide under a mushroom. Nevertheless, it was very nurturing my spiritual needs to communicate and exchange my thoughts, beliefs and my upbringing in the Israeli education system. I was clear about Sister Paula's life-style I so often tried to bring to her attention and awareness. It took me a while to realize how deeply her commitments and emotions were imbedded in her, yet evidently I never discovered its true depth. I had to learn that lesson by buffing my horns against the iron strong walls of brainwash. Since I am such a freethinker, it took my best energy and efforts to write rather than scream. So here is the reason.

I wished that throughout our philosophical communications, Sister Paula would open a tiny little slit in her concepts and dare to make a few changes by understanding how God is not out there, but in everyone and everything. I was wrong, and like Sister Paula, closed to believe that others can feel and believe to their death.

Chapter 3: Sudden Turn of Reality

Here my dear reader, Sister Paula and I are taking you through the very serious struggles any person would face when reality takes a major turn and the routine daily given in our life has to be altered as it had never before. Here we look into our own mirror as to how far we live in a bubble shaped not by our own decision-making and choices but by our peer pressure.

How much courage and power we need in order to overcome those elements that have been running our life, or, whether we cannot come up with that emotional, spiritual and physical energy to save our life. I have seen those conflicts time and again throughout my practice and the most extreme I found here with sister Paula, and decided to share it for each of us to look into our own mirror. If we chose life, and must understand that it is our life, and only we can live it.

August 16, 2007

Dear Dr. Yael,

I was going to answer your last e-mail when I found your beautiful gift of art.

Thank you for sending it to me, I really appreciated and enjoyed it immensely. I will explore the religious gallery too when my time allows me to enjoy it. Your last e-mail about your 'encounter' with Jesus was precious. After all, Jesus was born Jewish and so was his family and since you believe in destiny it may have been the right time in your life to meet him in a way you never had before. Thank you also for sharing your frustration with the bureaucracy and how interesting the end results were. I am happy for the father of your attorney. Yes, God is guiding us in ways that often are difficult for us to understand but his love is truthful and unvarying.

Now I would like to tell you my story that developed throughout this past week. I went to my annual physical check up to update our required health file given that we are working with children and disabled people, and as I mentioned a lump in my breast the doctor displayed deep concern, urging me to have it thoroughly checked, which I have. Tomorrow morning I am scheduled for a biopsy although the mammography and ultrasound exams clearly specify "highly malignant." His suggestion is "a very aggressive course of treatments," but I prefer to continue the natural and homeopathic approach under your guidance. My sisters in our covenant are very concerned and are oblivious of the homeopathic treatments. I printed from your website the link *Introduction to Simple Ways to Good Health* where you outline a treatment of prevention and healing for cancer; they read it but are still in doubt. I realize that their concern comes from love, certainly and especially Sr. Lucia, who is the oldest and the leader of our unity, and who feels the responsibility to take care of each of us in the best possible way she knows. I have not started yet to implement your suggestions of no animal proteins for the reason that they see it as too extreme a diet and fear it may cause potential health damage. My peers' pressure is powerful and demanding, although guided by love; it still lays very heavy on me. Please pray for me to make a God-guided decision, which is all I want.

Love and prayers,
Sister Paula

August 17, 2007

Dear Sister Paula,

Thank you for your e-mail. Here I am sending you the phone number of the skeptical attorney who said to me, "I owe you everything in the world. My father is with me and is getting better every day." Call her. She will be happy to share her thoughts and experience with you. Think of it as your body, your soul and your life. Cancer develops when we do not find the power and courage in us to adjust to our life circumstances and changes or when our immune system, as well as our approach and interaction with and toward our environment, is disabled or dysfunctional because we suppress it or because we feel we have no choice or we don't seem to find a way out of the situation, or even because we gave our "word" or our "oath" and fear to be blamed for walking out of the beaten path. Or when we don't seem to find any way to compensate our "little child" in us in a constructive and or creative exchange, or for any other reason. Even the absolute enclosure of every piece of your body for fifty years so no air and no sun can ever touch in your uniform, denies the so vital and necessary light and breath. Unable to address and resolve our fears or behavior patterns and instead, satisfy and 'please' others, rather than stand fast and acknowledge our own needs. We may act and handle our life in accordance or have the feeling that we "ran out of power" and so we live as we depleted our life force that we deny and never replenish—as annual vacations don't suffice. Or when we do not attend to our needs and wants and consistently fight them. Very typical for people who get lost in the jungle of outer demands upon them and lose contact with their inner truth. This so often happens to very religious individuals like nuns and monks, nurses and physicians, police and firefighters, mothers, outstanding good soldiers and employees. We must take a few moments for ourselves daily in order not to lose our connection with ourselves.

Even something so simple as the need to run to the bathroom, yet, circumstances do not 'allow' it. Like a schoolteacher who has to wait till the end of class, or a nurse or mother or bus driver—we all find ourselves in such situations. When these 'strain-full' situations are just temporary and not a usual way of life, it doesn't harm us, but if it is an ongoing life pattern, eventually it may harm.

Joan was a nurse I knew who worked night shifts for many years. She was in a group of ladies with whom we met weekly for beading. Every morning she would tell us how much coffee she had throughout the night and that she had not even a minute to go to the bathroom. She often declined fresh vegetable salads we brought for lunch because it was "too much foliage for me to stomach," she would say. Then, at the early age of sixty-three, she was diagnosed with bladder cancer. She said to me, "I can't understand why I got it. I was vegetarian and lived very healthy." If she had to deny her body rest at night, had too much coffee and denied her body the basic need and go to the bathroom, fresh vegetables were "too much foliage," she was in denial of her real health needs.

To "choke" us and deny the fresh and good energy flow including everything our soul and body need - creates blockages and eventually the body becomes very ill.

In order to resume health we have to remember that we are natural creatures. As such we have needs and necessities that must be addressed. Still, we were raised and trained to 'hold' our urine, 'hold' our feelings, repress and refrain our emotions, succeed at work no matter what, be a "good nun", a "good boy", "good wife" and "good employee". So are all the other different life avenues demand the best of us and exist like machines, cars, robots, and statues or maybe silk flowers. But not like the tree, bird or lizard. We have to obey social orders by the society in which we live. I don't suggest we turn into wild, unharnessed animals by any means. What I suggest is this: be aware of all those and find the golden path between your natural necessities and the right, appropriate order and discipline. They have to synchronize and be adjusted with us as natural creatures. There are hours, minutes, days we can take a break; like the Holy Sabbath by the Jewish tradition—even God took a break and rested on Sabbath.

This is when meditation comes in handy and vital. Our need for food is not valued higher than our need for rest and deep sleep, and water. Our need for sleep is not more important than our need to be listened to in order to express our thoughts and feelings—the way we do so is of our individual choice. All those needs must be attended and never denied.

You will be guided but please reflect prior to allowing your sister's lack of education, knowledge, experience and their ignorance, scare you and maybe even 'decide' for you. This attorney's mother had been a nurse and shared with us her forty years of practice with cancer patients in the hospital where she worked. She still appreciated the benefits of natural healing for her husband who agreed in spite of his skeptical feelings as well. The doctors sent him home to die since they exhausted their means in cancer therapy. He had been given every possible medication and the highest amount of radiations he could bare and the most and best chemotherapy their medicine books had to offer, yet with zero results. Did they ever talk to him as a human being and tried to address his feelings, or perhaps suggest a change of his diet? All he ate was oxtail soups and French fries. Did they ever ask him to talk about his reasons to be so hateful to himself? He was extremely self-destructive and did his utmost "best" to punish himself.

Note: Cancer is not a death sentence, but a signal the body sends in order for us to pay attention stating, "I cannot continue this way anymore. I am in distress. I cannot continue to function when you are completely in denial. I have had it." Our body signals prompt us and beg us to allow the changes that could help regenerate and recover our immune system and balance our life force, in order to heal and stay healthy. Only the chemotherapy, radiations and surgeries turn cancer so deadly because the mainstream medicine's true understanding and intent is the absolute opposite of the body's needs. Instead of empowering and recovering the self healing mechanism which is our immune system, the conservative medicine idea is to suppress it and literally wipe it out; they burn poison and mutilate the body, completely disregarding the soul, mind and the emotions. Rather the treatments put even more challenges and burdens on the already broken immune system since now the body has to channel all the healing power to the burns, the wounds, and to release the toxins and thus, the body lacks even more of the desperately needed attention, awareness and comfort it so desperately needs. When we "fight" cancer, in reality we actually fight ourselves because by the main stream medicine way, all we do is mask the desperation and pain of not just the body, but the mind, emotions and soul as well. We try then, to cover up the emotional hurt and hopelessness with more fear, more feeling out of control, more "no light at the end of the tunnel"—it seems like consoling a widow with a portion of arsenic. Would we ignore our little baby when it hurts, fears or cries? Nonetheless, we do so when the body signals the need for help, proper conditions, food, water or to be listened to, or when the individual needs an essential change in its life. So achingly that if no substantial amend is made, self-destruction, resignation to decay will be the only option left. Conversely, if we listen to our deepest truth and properly respond to our needs, stop suppressing even the cold or allergies, and if any part of our body or soul hurts, not to ignore and admit painkillers or anti suppressant, or antibiotics, or anti-inflammatory medications, the body can easily conquer cancer. The white blood cells then will consume the cancer cells once the immune system regained it's functionality and good, long lasting health can take up again.

My dear Sister, I know you will make the right choice. We both are aware of the better choices we have at our disposal, rather than just fall prey and be another victim of ignorance, of the one sided approach of modern "sophisticated medicine" and pharmaceutical companies' 'research.' By choosing and refusing to be their 'poison consumer' for their own monetary benefits and lack of knowledge, which will lead to their wealth but to your death like so millions each year worldwide for many decades and still do.

Wait, it is not just greed and ignorance—the main stream medicine representatives are scared of the ramifications for their careers if they will not go by the books and by the institutes and FDA rules and regulations. The FDA—Federal Drug Administration—was originally assigned to protect the US citizens.

Almost funny had it not been very frightening and scary. Our own government kills us—it is the law.

Blessings and do not fear. Follow the light and it will show you the right way.

Yours,

Yael

August 18, 2007

Dear Sister Paula,

Since I do care and know the paths your community would like you to stride on I would like to share with you a little story over and above my thoughts. I am not sure that it will change your mind and lead you in a different direction but at least in front of the universe and God, I need the peace of mind knowing I have done my very best to convey this knowledge to you so you may make the best decision. In one of your previous emails you wrote how mysterious our acquaintance felt to you. Well maybe this is the true revelation for you?! Maybe this is one of our lessons and enlightenments to help us understand the reason behind our enigmatic connection.

In my first year in the USA I had a dear friend in Seattle. We knew each other since we met in Israel and later on even worked together. She would consult with me or send me her clients of different and very complicated neurological cases, and together we reached significant results. One day she referred to me a seventy-three-year old lady hoping I could help heal her as she was diagnosed with breast cancer. Apparently that lady was very concerned and frightened, as we all would be, with such a diagnosis. She called and told me how she had found me through my friend and asked if it was necessary for her to come and see me as I lived in Colorado at that time and she was, as I mentioned, in Seattle, Washington.

The idea that we could discuss everything over the phone made her at first a little apprehensive to say the least, and yet was a big relief for her on the other hand. To not have to travel away from home for each consultation took a huge burden and stress off her shoulders. I explained to her my approach to health, which is simple and natural opposed to the western medicine's way, and that I am not God and not every case is a sheer success. At times it takes more effort on the mental or the spiritual or even the social plain in order to achieve full recovery for many years. She took my advice and started a thirty-day vegetable juice fast. She shared with me that it was not easy for her, yet she preferred it to surgery and chemotherapy that offered such gloomy results in the end anyway. After thirty days she called me and said she felt very good and could not find her lump anymore. That lady returned to her doctor and underwent another thorough check up, which included a mammogram and ultrasound. To the doctor's surprise he could find no trace of cancer in her breast. Low and behold, though it was a good reason to celebrate she sounded shocked and was bitterly sobbing while on the phone with me. She tried to comprehend how the same doctor with the identical medical instruments and the same tests could not find the tumor anymore. With one strange exception: Unlike at the time of diagnosis, this time he found it inconceivable and was in disbelief and did not even trust in his own testing machines. She was still inconsolable as she was telling me about her doctor's responses to the test.

"He said it is absolutely impossible that a malignant tumor would disappear. We must do a biopsy," he said to her.

The same words I just now said to you I asked her: "Is it your life, your body and your decision or his?" But she, like you, mentioned to me the massive peer pressure from her family and friends and so she went for the biopsy. Well, dear Sister, will I let you guess what they found? They found nothing, which did not make the situation any easier on that lady. I assumed that at that point she would be very happy and would even celebrate her clean bill of health. But my assumption was wrong. The doctor as well as her family continued to put more pressure on her. And as the doctor assured them how important that procedure was for her, she gave her consent to having a mastectomy.

But, guess what they found? You guessed it... nothing. So my understanding is that if we succumb to peer pressure and ignorance we may even lose a few of our body parts or even worse, we give away the right to make our own decisions for our body, soul, mind and life. We may be seriously harmed mutilated and deformed for just one purpose: To succumb to and please the peers, the family and the doctors, and follow the mainstream, old-fashioned, long outdated dogma. My question is: Why don't we follow and go with nature? Why don't we allow the body to heal itself? Or, why don't we look around and see how many millions still die of cancer, yet know that in reality they don't die of cancer but they all die of the cancer 'therapy' rather than the cancer itself. Haven't we seen it every day for the past centuries? Don't we all know by now that it is not about fighting cancer, but about the many billions of dollars in revenue made by the medical industry, all together? Is it not clear that we have to choose whether we are willing to be their prey or their finance source, or rather neither but simply save our lives? Do we consent to die for them so they do not lose their license or job because they derail from 'the books' and "hospital guidelines and policy" and actually use their own judgment and understanding of health properties and treasures? Or are we ready to sacrifice our precious life for the sake of 'being good' or 'being easy to get along with' or 'being obedient' or 'not being rebellious or a trouble maker' or may be we should just die and not swim against the stream? Or all of the above.

My dear Sister, one thing you know for sure: I don't get rich off your health care. I treat you for the good turn of your health and my own conscious. So my agenda can never be suspected as untrue, insincere or for greed only. Not even for my ego, since the success in healing cancer is not applied to my credit but to the natural self-healing mechanisms you were born with. Here is a web site you should read before you make your final decision: www.cancertutor.com.

Thank you for being another important lesson in my life.

Yours,

Yael

August 23, 2007

Dear Dr. Yael,

Thank you, thank you with all my heart for your e-mail from August 17th, and your strong answer regarding the course of action I should take confronting my cancer. Deep in my heart and mind I felt that this is the way to follow and your encouragement gave me more peace and strength to convince all the others. My sisters accepted my decision and will support me in following it in any way possible. Also, our Dr. accepted it without imposing any more pressure on me. He was very surprised and said he never heard about a natural way for treating cancer. I talked to him yesterday when he gave me the results of the biopsy, which confirms the findings of the mammography. I told him to look at the web site you pointed out to me, it may be an education he needs.

Now what shall I do? I must admit that with all that I read I am a little confused. How will you direct me? And shall I come and see you? Or can you tell me what to do by e-mail? I trust the purity of your intentions; I have full confidence in you as a doctor and as a person who is full of compassion and faith. You can certainly not make a fortune taking care of me but it should not be done completely free for the sake of justice. My community accepts my decision and offers to support me financially as well as needed and as is possible. I would like to ask you so many little practical questions, even as simple as where to buy my vegetables. I will have to find the time to incorporate my meeting for treatments with you into my very busy schedule and my responsibilities, and I am not sure it will be possible on a regular basis.

I may sound silly but please be patient. I will wait to hear from you in peace and in prayers. At night I can sit at the computer and enjoy the beautiful pictures of Israel, or of the art galleries; thank you, thank you again for sending them to me, they have been an unexpected gift bringing spiritual joy and enlightenment.

Keeping you in my love and prayers,

Sister Paula

August 24, 2007

Dear Sister Paula,

And I thank the universe for your decision. Well, the most important part is: To learn how important you are on this planet and how your soul has been crying out for your attention and care for so long. This is the most important part in your healing process. However, please read again your last email in which you write: " I will have to find the time to incorporate my meeting for treatments with you into my very busy schedule and my responsibilities, and I am not sure it will be possible on a regular basis." Read it as many times as possible to understand how you like to heal, but cannot take the time for it, since your schedule and responsibility still take first priority in your perception. Sorry, but this is a worrisome start for "change" in order to heal. I don't really know how to approach a nun and convince her to take care of herself more than all the others she has under her care, and how can I help her learn the value of her own life? We have to tackle this subject seriously, knowing how this will probably be your main obstacle on your path to true health. I don't intend to argue with religion. My understanding is that before God, good health and happiness is our basic and foremost born right regardless of our core beliefs. Rest and sleep must also be a major component in healing, recovering and reactivating your immune system. Please take it seriously into your consideration. It doesn't sound very promising and determined and committed to making the needed changes for your own health when you say, "I will have to find the time to incorporate my meetings for treatments with you into my very busy schedule and my responsibilities and I am not sure it will be possible on regular basis." You will have to make time for your treatments and understand the importance of the changes you have to make in order to heal and live. Natural healing is about taking responsibility for our own health versus the so-called 'traditional' medicine that takes that responsibility for us and from us—no changes—are only in death.

The vegetables you will be using must be organic. Get yourself a juicer for a minimum of five glasses of vegetable juice per day, preferably one of those that leaves the pulp and does not separate and waste it. You may feel a little weak the first few days, which requires more rest as this is really the best time for meditation and prayer and a time for more relaxation. Drink as much water as possible, and yes, purified water would be the best option. Clean water is vital for better health. Please get yourself a bottle of organic apple cider vinegar, which can be purchased at any health food store or any food store. The important vegetables to juice are: carrots, celery and kale, collard greens, beets with leaves, sweet potatoes and green apple, spinach leaves and parsley, sugar snaps and green peas, broccoli and lemon with its white and yellow peel, bell pepper and a little bit of garlic, ground flax seeds, chia seeds and nutritional yeast. You can combine the ingredients according to your own taste preferences. The Pulse Electromagnetic Field Therapy device must be incorporated since it supports and activates the healthy cells functions to regain their efficient metabolism in order to enhance and vitalize your immune system. The Pulsed Electromagnetic Therapy promotes relaxation and supports your body to bind and absorb significantly more oxygen as well as nutrients. The cancer cells become 'devastated' by those cancer adverse 'new conditions' your body will start to develop, and since the cancer cells can thrive only in a very low immune system environment, and cannot exist in a healthy environment that provides the healthy cells needs, the 'poor' cancer cells gradually die off and be consumed by the body as foreign proteins, consumed and wasted by the expelling organs, like the kidney and intestines.

To my understanding this is certainly a significantly better way than any chemotherapy because the chemotherapy is killing the immune system instead of recovering and strengthening it. This should be helped and supported by the Pulsed Electromagnetic Field Therapy, by healthy cell nutrition, as well as a healthy and a balanced lifestyle, some kind of daily exercise that is gentle and not strenuous, and through paying higher respect to the true natural needs of the body and soul. Changing our state of mind to a more positive responsible view of life and happy attitude. Responsible; I mean responsible to your own health and life and not just responsible for others. (The latter leave to God. It is His or Her job, not yours.) Yes, you will need plenty of rest, positive thinking, and if you could see me once or twice a week it would be helpful for your body and the mental and emotional as well. We could also exchange e-mail if you prefer, however they will not serve your entire needs on your path to recovery because healing and rest is an important part of your change of priorities. To take time for yourself, to leave the responsibility to your other sisters as you need to restore the Goddess in you and reclaim your right to health and life. I guess this would be the whole secret. You have made a good choice that takes work and self-discipline; nevertheless, it is a beautiful journey after all. It is your journey in and unto life. This time the journey is of your own life. God bless you.

Remember that God gave you a clear signal that you are the most important now rather than your schedule!

Yours,

Yael

August 26, 2007

Dear Dr. Yael,

I still have to take the first step on this "beautiful journey" you defined for me and to be completely honest with you I must say: I am scared and hope you can help me. But please don't think of me as a special person for being a nun. I am a woman, weak and confused, and at this point questioning if my decision was really following God's will or was my first wish, to ignore completely this lump, not a better way of letting God take its course without any human interference. The part that scares me most is the fasting time, how long can it be? I am not retired although I am seventy-three years old and have a lot of energy, so shall I retire now? Shall I take a leave of absence? Or may I continue my work with the children only part time incorporating the time I need for rest and healing? I know that life is more important than a schedule but what shall I preserve my life for if doing nothing? And what if I will be weak, shaking and hungry? Will I not be able even to pray or meditate?

The other difficulty I see is to find the products you listed. I located a health food store not too far and purchased the organic vinegar and the stevia. They did not have the stevia in liquid form but only a powder. I have not yet found a place to buy the organic vegetables. I live in a very poor neighborhood where I cannot find any organic vegetables. There is a supermarket with organic food not too far but the variety of vegetables is very limited and packed in small packages of 4 oz. How many vegetables do I need to get five glasses of juice per day? Can you please indicate the name of some stores where I can find the organic vegetables in the amount and variety I need? I am sorry if I aggravate you with my questions. I trust you as a doctor and as a messenger of God's will and this is the only reason for not giving up my decision.

Love,

Sister Paula

August 27, 2007

Dear Sister Paula,

Your concerns are very natural and understandable, and who can blame you? After all, this is not just a new diet or a retirement but a whole new approach to yourself, your health, your life and the relations between you and your environment. Even between yourself, your convent and God. I don't think that God's intention is to see you suffer by getting weak or sicker. I feel that this is part of your physical and soul's journey and learning adventure, which should be a beholden, grateful and very empowering journey. I can sense how it brings you the closest to God as you have ever been because it is your first time in life to fully comprehend and serve the concept of "God created us in his own image." Therefore we must respect our life, our health and our well-being like we do respect him. And remember you mentioned you're born sister and asked God to take care of her, because for all others it is well his job, only for you it is solely your job and responsibility.

We walk a certain path our entire life until we realize that we arrived at a dead end, just like you did with your health or others may in their many different life avenues, like failing businesses or relationships or even incarceration. In your case you have lost your good health and vitality as your body breaks down. Here we are forced to make decisions and change the path we had been surely striding for so long. Sometimes it is a good one and we find a better place and sometimes it can be a lesser path. Life is full of the decisions we must make yet fear is weakening us more than anything. Like Churchill said: "The only thing one must fear is fear itself."

Hence cancer is not a death sentence; it forces us to pave new directions to a better outcome. Cancer is not an indication of chemotherapy, deficiency or surgery deprivation, or the shortness of radiation either; on the contrary, cancer is a clear indication of a major breakdown of our auto immune system for certain reasons, mostly to be found inside us and not outside of our own life. When cancer implies the body lost control over its immune system, it is the turning point in which we realize that our health balance in our 'health bank' reached an all-low point. Is this a time to just cut the 'bank account' out and run away or burn the bank? (same as the cancer treatment of mainstream medicine) I see those solutions as doomed to fail if we understand the need to restore our balance, our true and long lasting health balance. Consequently we need to learn, (like with our bank account), to spend less of our resources, and earn more vitality by better care and check where the energy money goes. If we burn the bank it will only bring us to a worse state. Hence the same idea pertains to our health. We all develop cancer cells at certain points in our lives and our immune system always detects and consumes them, regarding them as foreign proteins that have no business in our body and forces them to "commit suicide" by consuming the cancer cells with lymphatic and white blood cells, by phytochemicals, and oxygen enriched blood, healthy food causing the weak cancer cells to collapse.

Accordingly the most important point is to look at the cancer cells for what they truly are. They are weak cells that developed in error of the protein chains when the healthy cells temporarily lost control, and they have no connection to the brain like our own healthy cells have. Each healthy cell that belongs to the body's functions is controlled and connected to the 'body control tower,' which the cancer cells don't belong to. Nevertheless if we deny them their 'comfort zone' by depriving them of the proper conditions they need for thriving, they will simply die off. This is the battle for our life for as long as we live the ongoing combat between the 'good and evil.' Cancer cells love sugars of all kinds, they love acidic environment just like the fungi and as many of us don't realize that athlete's foot is fungi, and instead of using all those miraculous anti fungal medications, sprays and creams, they would be much better off had they alkaline their blood consistency by enriching the blood with oxygen. Then, oops, the fungi die. So simple. Stress, sleep deprivation, fast food, baked goods, alcohol, etc. are fungi and cancer favoring conditions because they all create over acidity, which cancer cells thrive on.

Same in the world surrounding us, it is in our own body. As the garden flowers need the proper conditions to bloom, without them they will die. Every living cell has to have the ideal conditions in order to thrive and only under those absolute proper conditions can they live. Yet if denied them, they will die. The body creates and builds cancer cells in times of desperation and dysfunction and when denied the proper conditions for good health and a strong immune system, however, when the body stops the detriment conditions and resumes good and healthy conditions for its functional immune system, those cancer cells will die off. They suddenly do not get what they really need for thriving and multiplying. These cancer cells (like bacteria, fungi and viruses) suddenly get overloaded with large amounts of oxygen, which by itself kills them, and also when they suddenly receive surfeit anti oxidant rich foods rather than toxic food. Suddenly the environment becomes alkaline instead of acidic and that also is unbearable for cancer cells, the immune system grows gradually stronger and 'throws' the negative equilibrium 'out of balance' and restores the positive vital equilibrium.

As you understand, my dear Sister, I would not suggest succumbing to the evil because "I fear it" or because "I am afraid to fight it," but because I understand and make my educated and intelligent choice. For your entire adult life you have been obedient and selfless. You have done your utter best for all the people you have been working with. You have been at service to your community and sisters for so many years. Now is your turn to step up for your own life and reclaim it. You should not be scared to fight and 're-educate' your own body and modify your patterns to resume life. The question you asked, "What is life for if we cannot work, serve, and pray," is the most important issue that may be also your biggest hurdle on your way to recovery.

Why can't we see life simply for what it is? Life! To get up in the morning and thank God for seeing the light, for smelling the fresh air and seeing the beautiful flowers, for the water we drink and shower in, and for our breath pumping in our lungs? Was God conditioning our first breath by our service to him and the public or prayers? Does God stipulate our life by suffering, illness and despair? Or if it is true that God created us in his own image he also gave us the abundance of his world! Do you truly believe that God is there for himself or his creations for suffering? Well, Jesus was a human being who thought he should take the worlds sufferings upon himself, but if he did so then does it not mean that you and I are saved by him and are now free to embrace life for its goodness, abundance and joy?

Sure work and serving, of course, too yet if we do not respect our health, how can we serve and transmit healthy energy? Will the wheel not turn then and we will have to be served? Is there anything I don't understand here? Is there something you would like to explain that proves your rightful path to health and happiness is somehow wrong or sinful?

Personally, I can't help but see the correlation between the 'victim' types with cancer or cardiac disease and even liver and chronic intestinal illnesses. Because "Auto-Immune-System" means "Self-Help System" and therefore it must be cultivated in all aspects of our life. Cancer means "No Self-Help System" in office. Victims do not have the power to fight the adversity whether is it a disease, an enemy or social situation in which we simply should not succumb or give in. Some people are known to be in control of their family, or friends or even country, yet have no control over their own body and life. This is the point we must grow out of and mature from and learn that "I" can only be in control over my own life, and when "I" fail to do so "I" get very ill.

On the other hand, when trying and take control over others, disregarding our own life necessities, we set ourselves up to become very sick as well. So the key is to realize that we cannot control anyone else's life but only our own. Hence the name "Auto-Immune-System" says it all. Nonetheless, it is not only about our blood consistency, the vitamin indications or our liver and intestines. Our anger control skills and how far we let it sink into our life, our self-defense mechanism. The clear boundaries we set between the negative impact of the environment surrounding us at times—this Immune System refers also to our adaptability; it is about our barriers and control over our thoughts, memories and the way we learn to handle them. We must learn how to channel negative memories or hardship from the past into healthy creative and positive actions. When I was in the midst of sadness and turmoil in my life, I was each day on the tennis court and in my painting room after work. This is what life is all about—life is about entirely *all* and *everything*. Do you see chemotherapy or surgery capable of transforming the whole picture of health, life and thinking? Since life is so precious and has been given to you for the one and only purpose of living, per se. Please ask yourself what God's Will truly is?

In the Jewish tradition as we celebrate Yom Kippur, we are obliged to ask forgiveness of anyone we may have hurt somehow on our path, whether accidentally or in rage, and when we don't we may not be forgiven by God and not be written in His book of life. What it actually means is this: if we cannot apologize to others and forgive ourselves for our mistakes we torture our own soul and sicken our physical plane, which leads to disease. It is a very advanced social value to be able to forgive others, yet given the notion that we are all one and that we are created in his image, consequently we have to set ourselves free of guilt, anger or any other negative feelings in order to heal and prevail.

Only when we are free of hate, resentment, fear, jealousy, unsatisfied, ungrateful, rage, and all the other negative emotions, can we then appreciate the bliss of life, as it says: "In our heart and our soul." Even the ancient thinkers knew the correlation between the body and soul. Why the orthodox medicine doesn't know and recognize this connection is still a puzzle to me.

Why would anyone dare to ridicule God's intelligence, the almighty ruler of the whole universe, the sun and the stars and all that is above and beyond by thinking he or she doesn't understand it? And for the reason that life is time limited and will eventually end for everyone. Even Jesus lived and died. No one is immortal. The question is not when do we die but when and how do we live. We, you and I, have been doing the best to our understanding in order to please, whether it is god, people, community, family, boss, superior or children, hence are we aware of the important responsibility we carry in us to maintain in a pleasing manner the sanctuary God has given us for our own soul to reside in. Your cancer is 'whispering' into your ear, "Don't take life for granted and do not miss out even one day of your life. Live your life; be attentive and grateful for every breath you take, for each ray of the sun, for every taste and good smell, for every drop of rain and twit of the bird. Do not ignore and do not take it ever for granted because it has been given to you as a gift; it is literally your present. Be in this world and only present actions lead to the better future."

So my answer is: juice-fasting doesn't make you weak, the healing process makes you tired, as the body needs the energy to utilize and waste bad food we do not need. While you fast your cells receive pure, 'healthy cell's food' and can become only healthier and stronger cells.

I want to remind you how people in poor countries eat little, stay slim and strong, and suffer significantly less of the known degenerative diseases our modern society faces resulting from overeating and indulgence. The juice fasting should last, if possible, thirty days though the majority of people start to feel a lot better after the first 3-5 days. Throughout the juice fast you will need to drink plenty of water and lots of rest in order to help your body heal and preserve its energy for you intention to heal, rather than any other purpose. Sure, you may get tired depending mainly upon your attitude and energy management.

If you keep on praying remember the appreciation of the opportunity you have been granted to open your eyes and make all the necessary changes in your life in order to live. This is the time to apply all those life modifications and life conditions to your desperate needs rather than adjust your needs to your life demands solely—anymore.

You probably are going to enjoy even more energy than you presently have and perhaps feel notably better in the resurrection and restoration of your soul and body sanctuary. The same as you would feel joyous for the neatness and cleanliness of a sacred sanctuary so you will feel proud, happy, grateful and empowered to participate on your journey to recovery. Treating our soul's sanctuary as such is our number one responsibility. All these aspects of your life have probably been overlooked by you for too long and must undergo major restitution, purification and repair and must be treated with respect and gratitude just like the holy places to which we come to meet and be the closest with God. The idea is to be accountable for our own life, body and health and this means meeting God in us every moment of our being. Just like rodents and mice hate clean, neat and cultivated places, so do the cancer cells 'hate' the "junk-free" healthy body conditions. The healthy cells get more power and full of zip when they start to reclaim the reign over our body and mind, for our most sacred asset, life. This is a magnificent process that you don't want to miss.

In regards to your questions where to find fresh produce in your area, I am not familiar with your neighborhood and this is also part of your journey by taking matters into your own hands and caring for the quality of food you serve yourself for your own health. This is your duty for your own life. From then on, after you started your juice fasting and if you are able to work again, do it. Be attentive and responsive to your body's signals, listen to yourself and if you need more rest – Rest. The world will continue to find solutions even if you and I are not here to help 'save' it anymore. So we need to take charge and be liable and responsible for our well-being in order not to fall burden on those we have been trying to serve and save our entire life. On the whole, the most important issue for you now is if you need to take a break, take it. Prayers need no more power or energy than what we already have. We don't need a special place and time to pray, we can do it everywhere and at any time.

Detoxifying doesn't make us weaker although we may feel a little tired only for a short time, but it sure empowers us. Don't we know about the importance of recommended fasts by all religions? Wise ancient cultures advocate the less and simpler foods and fasts increase the healing properties and clears the mind, residues and waste pollute the body and soul, and the energy necessary to waste and struggle with the overloads, is saved and turns into energy the body uses to preserve health and life and regenerates the well functioning Auto Immune System. Fasting is the best cleansing and best antibiotic nature has.

I hope you understand my e-mail and that this will guide you on your precious new voyage. This is the condensed work of *Body, Mind and Spirit*. See, even a nun ought to learn that she was born not merely help others but to facilitate her self as well. Because if she will keep herself well, her ability to serve God's Will and be strong for others will be enhanced and she will be able to serve the real self in her rather than be deprived, which consequently will cause her to become burden on her congregation as a sick and helpless person.

Good health for you means; that you could be an excellent role model for your congregation, show more respect to God, and find gratitude and appreciation for life. The more people who understand this concept and follow, the better our entire world will become.

Think about it. We are made of about 90% water. Water consists of molecules that have an electromagnetic field just like everything else. The many water molecules are exactly the same as what we are made of and like every flower, every tree or butterfly, every lake, ocean and river is made of. Imagine how the purity depends upon the molecule's purity and about all the creatures in the ocean, the rivers and lakes and how we all are dependent upon the single molecule's purity and balance.

The same goes for our health. Each molecule in our body has to function well and be intact in order to maintain the whole body's health and function at its top performance. Just like the oceans cleanliness impacts and influences the livelihood of everything, so must we realize that the same rules apply to us as well.

Healthy molecules make healthy cells and healthy cells make healthy organs, and impact the healthy mind and spirit, which in turn creates, keeps, maintains and balance good overall health. That has the 'contagious' effect upon our family, our community and congregation, and the complete world.

Believe it or not, this actually creates a healthy earth. Consequently, allow me to say that the better you, I, and all the other people who take care of others, the better we may be able to contribute to the vast ocean of health and love.

This is how the secret of one nun's good health works. One nun, one child, one woman, one man, one water molecule—this is how it works.

A healthy world is undoubtedly a better peaceful and loving place to live in. The secret for a healthier planet is not just in our safe sanctuary of churches, synagogues and temples, but also in each of us. We all can contribute to the universe's best.

Blessings,

Yael

Reflections

Listen to your deepest truth—this is the first step to healing. Is it sinful to seek health in a natural way and take responsibility to our own health? Is this what God wants? Or are God's servants trying to convince us not to make the effort to live a healthy life?

Peer pressure plays a powerful role in many of us, but we are supposed to listen to our inner voice, not fearful voices speaking from ignorance and fear rather than intelligence and education. Paula's concerns about the dangers of homeopathy are unfounded, but her doctors and peers shared her fears, which made it very difficult for her to let her body heal itself. Paul's friends and doctors were ignoring the fact that many millions still die of cancer in spite of the advanced science and research. The only danger in homeopathy is if the homeopath doesn't know what s/he is doing, and still then, it cannot damage like wrong surgery, wrong medications, etc. Consider how mild the risk of homeopathy is as compared to more invasive medicine. It is true that if we chose the juicing method to heal, we may feel weak for a while, but is the juice is weakening us? My answer is this: juice fasting doesn't make you weak, the healing process makes you tired; the body needs the energy to utilize and waste bad food we do not need.

It is also critical to note that Sister Paula denied herself constructive attention to her inner child. Her live was almost completely void of playing or fun, and she limited her air and sunshine. Her smile, happiness, joy, light, and breath were unnecessarily restricted by her asceticism and hardship. In spite of her fear of her frightening diagnosis, Sister Paula could not find the time to heal. This is not the way to natural health. It shows how she could not really make the necessary shift to seek and achieve better health. Why didn't Paula do what it takes—devote the requisite time and effort—to allow the body to heal itself?

We all must learn to be loyal and attentive to our inner truth unlike the strict disciplines as in the convent, military, or the Queen's Guards. If we deny our being, our need for love, joy, and comfort, which are absolutely vital for our existence, we plant the seeds for illness, depression, anger, and other emotions that can make us sick. Then we seek the best medications to suppress the symptoms of our illness, and so our immune system collapses at a certain point and cancer cells start to encapsulate, and eventually a tumor is formed.

When we "fight" cancer, in reality we actually fight ourselves. Illness will develop at the most vulnerable and neglected part of the body (whether physical or emotional), or the part that represents suppressed functionality and vitality. Like breasts and uterus in nuns, or prostate cancer in priests, or liver cancer in angry and depressed individuals and so on.

When the doctor gives the cancer diagnosis to his/her patient, s/he can't see any hope other than a long and painful course of treatment that may or may not be effective, and we all dread those words: "you have cancer of the...." and we hear "no light at the end of the tunnel," and every function in the body starts to shut down. But read again this marvelous story of that lady in Seattle, Washington. Although she succumbed to her family's pressure and allowed the doctor to act on his doubts and badly injure her, she still healed.

Cancer is not a death sentence. However, it forces us to pay better attention to our natural needs and satisfy them in order to achieve a better outcome. We must realize that cancer cells need a very specific environment in order to exist, and if they don't have it, they die out and are consumed by our immune system. Every creature in nature that needs its specific life conditions—if it doesn't have them it will die. When we embrace homoeopathic methods, we nurture an environment in our bodies where cancer cannot survive.

A *cancer survivor* is every person who accepts the message from his or her body and makes fundamental changes in his or her physical, emotional, social and spiritual life.

Chapter 4: Loving Yourself

Loving God is completely misinterpreted by many religious leaders. Sacrifice and deprivation of nuns and other believers doesn't bring them closer to God, because we cannot love when we starve, suffer, and deny ourselves. The failures of the church are reflected in the poor health of those who are most dedicated to serving God.

In chapter four we see cracks in Paula's trust in her views of mainstream medicine. She begins to better embrace homeopathy, but she still has the same old doubts that hold her back and handicap her ability to enjoy the rewards of good health. She still clings to God and her doctors (including myself) rather than depending on and listening to her own inner voice. If she had done so, she would have realized her freedom to feel and grasp divinity without any church or bishop.

We cannot ignore our inner voice and avoid or deny our needs; otherwise, our lives will always end in tragedy. This is why no researched results and consequences can be accurate as long as the research objective ignores the needs of the inner self.

August 29, 2007

Dear Dr. Yael,

Thank you very much again for your prompt response, for your encouragement and for the charge of moral strength and clear ideas that transpire from all your words. For me it is really a soul searching time; I based all my life on the moral principle that "to be" is more important than "to do" and now I am faced with the reality of applying it and yet – I tremble. Please keep praying for me. On the practical level I made a little progress with my sisters' help. We found good vegetables at a big market and we also bought the juicer. So I am ready to start but have two more questions: How big should each glass be? In regards to the pulp, do you suggest I drink or eat it or toss it? Please bear with me and understand how inexperienced I am in handling all the details.

"Seek first the Kingdom of God and His justice and all these things shall be given you besides," says the Gospel, and "these things" is everything that comes with life and everything that we may hope for now and forever.

May God Bless You, with love and thankfulness—
Sister Paula

August 30, 2007

Dear Sister Paula,

Trembling and shaking is part of the survival instinct, especially when we enter the unknown and face life threatening situations, fear for our life or when we are controlled by our dread and anxiety. It happens also when our feeding habits change and we stop consuming high sugars, coffee, baked goods, etc. The leading difference between my approach to health and that of mainstream is the placing of control over our health and life into our own hands. I am a big advocate of hope and positive thinking and helping the challenged and ill see the light at the end of the tunnel though not through a series of toxic and killing medicine, as you know by now, but by taking the needed actions to apply and alter the necessary in our life in order to resume vitality and well-being. Our cells are like little children. When you tell them, "You are going to die," they hear the message and prepare to shut down and die. However, if you tell them, "You are strong, you can and

112

will overcome the adversity and see how much fun is awaiting you," they will "get their act together" and will shift into the idea that, "Hey, look how much fun is awaiting you!"

That is the huge difference between hope and hopelessness. The same difference between a fun and joy seeking child and a grumpy negative and hopeless old person. It is the same difference seen between light at the end of the tunnel, and no light at all. We must always tune into light.

I would never pile the bad news on any of my patients when the lab tests results return regardless how hopeless they appear to be. What I will and always do is guide the individual to the many different options to regenerate and recover good and balanced health. The fear and anxiety crop up when a person listens to the doctor's gruesome news, which makes them feel helpless and totally out of control. How evil is it to be so discourteous instead of being supportive and guide the individual into an active and assertive journey on their so needed health. To teach every person the many different avenues he or she can take in order to help the crashed immune system regain its vital force and get back on track. As you now understand there are numerous good options we can choose from on our path to the glory by winning the battle of resurrection and reclaim our good health.

To tremble and fear is natural when obtaining that bad news from your doctor.

Hence, up until now you have been relying on the traditional and familiar way of life as suddenly your life takes this major shift forcing you to face a new situation, oblige you to modify and replace the old with the new, the known with the unknown and different so you can pave the path to win back your life.

Unexpectedly you are called to assume responsibility for your own life and well-being. It probably feels to you like dying. It is very scary in every culture and at every age. Nonetheless as you had taken the oath to serve and obey the Church's rules and regulations as well as the covenant and never to question or doubt, just follow and pray, you handed all responsibilities for your well-being, life, body, mind and spirit to that which you committed yourself to for your entire life. In the past five years since we met you clearly experienced a shift in your view of life. Your anger and disappointments at the management clashed with your values and beliefs, significantly enough to the point where you realized the impact it had upon your health. When talking about your struggles, your whole being flushed of anger and of your deep disillusionment as I remember. I believe that every nun in your sisterhood has gone through similar emotional times. You started a very deep change in your existence, which is what led us to cross our paths. Now your soul is taking you to the next level – taking conscientiousness for yourself as you are learning the importance of your private well-being.

Unlike the life you had lived for the past fifty years, knowing and strongly believing that your work and service were and still are always your first priority. The trembling and anxiety in part are your body's survival instincts and the other part is the brainwashing, one of your guilt for inhibited functionality for the healing time, and second, that cancer is a final death sentence. Little do we know that cancer is the 'loudest cry' of the body, the soul and mind for radical transformation, and things such as food, nutrition and a mundane life style are just the tip of the iceberg. As you said, "Do the soul search." Please do not fear death, but instead search for life. Only when we give up on our basic life necessities will life be replaced by death.

See, the balance is the most important issue throughout life. To be only greedy and corrupt is creating disease, as well as to be totally submissive and absolutely obedient to a total non-material lifestyle (which even you started to realize is not so non-materialistic as we would like to continue to believe) and with the absolute selflessness and acquiescence to the congregation's demands and regulations on the other hand, are another way of imbalance. We are made of all: material body, esoteric mind and spirit, feelings, needs, necessities, desires, lust and ego. Every one of us has to search for the balance and restore it in order to avoid getting sick. This, my love, is what you are doing now. And if so, please don't put all the emphasis on the juicer, juicing and pulp and on all the material and practical changes alone. Live, smell, be grateful for every drop of juice. Only life can give life. Good thoughts create good things; start to find joy, smile, and create your own inner happiness. Healthy thoughts bring health. This is the closest we can get to God on the spiritual and material level; this is the physical part of us. On the material level by eating and drinking the wonderful nutrients God created for us, feeding your healthy cells with the same light that made the natural food grow like a tiny flashlight that is put into each and every cell in us. Because unhealthy cells cannot thrive and grow in the same healthy and lighted environment where the healthy cells thrive. Every vegetable you allow into your body is created by the magnificent interaction between light and water and they are precious creations of the universe, just like you, I, and everyone else. Bless them before you drink them and guide their good healing energy to enlighten your cells within, because that alone can bring the smile in your face and joy and happiness into your soul.

So my answer to your questions is: the amount and sizes are totally up to your desire and ability to drink it. It is very tasty and filling and you will see how you will not be hungry and how you will slowly build a beautiful stamina, one that you probably have long forgotten could reside in your body, mind and soul. My suggestion to you is use the glass or cup you like the most. (Every time you look at the juice see God and bliss. Smile!) In case you don't like to eat or drink the pulp it can be used for soups or compost piles if you have anything like that in your yard. Jewish observers bless every glass of water nearing their lips and every piece of food they eat. Water, like us, is very sensitive to intentions and prayers. The molecules change completely when exposed to good music, prayers and positive feelings. Every cup of vegetables holds God's (yours) highest intention for your health – bless it and be cheerful. Don't we all know that life is a journey? Embrace it. And please keep in mind that your journey is not just about the body and food, it is about your soul, feelings, thoughts, habits, beliefs. Only the collection of all that is you, your life and your attention and awareness to it, will pave the path to your complete health. This is what cancer truly is all about. If you think that juicing will solve all your problems, you may be unpleasantly surprised. It is not the lack of juice and pulp that brought you to your health breakdown to begin with.

Love,

Yael

September 5, 2007

Dear Dr. Yael,

Today I am on day four on my journey and I cannot find the words to describe how I feel. One word could be that I am "surviving." It is a time of prayer, yes, and of penance, but I am certainly far from the glorious feeling you described in your last email. I am not hungry at all but I am very weak, my legs are shaking all the time and I am always cold. My community is supporting me in every way possible but they also have questions. I would like to see you one time so we can talk better than we can through email so I may ask you all my questions and receive your answers directly. Please let me know when I can see you. Now I feel closer to Jesus on the cross; in a small way I am sharing his suffering and I don't want this time to be wasted but to be fully lived.

With love and prayers,

Sister Paula

September 7, 2007

Dear Dr. Yael,

I am now on my sixth day of the journey and did not receive any words from you, so I am sending my email again. Maybe something did not work right on the computer connection. I am coming along just the same. Thank you for your patience; please do not abandon me.

Love and blessings,

Sister Paula

September 12, 2007

Dear Sister Paula,

I am very proud of you for choosing the natural way to heal, which is not easy, yet unlike the mainstream way (detoxifying is putting a lot of strain and effort on the body, just like house cleaning)—safe. Your weakness is understandable and natural. You are not used to sugar baking goods and animal protein free juice-fasting as healing is strenuous on our body and requires more rest. Yet, this new adventure and challenge is tapping into the unknown world of self discipline for you, as you could not refrain from the sugar loaded cakes and 'substantial food' like meat, fish, potatoes and pasta, which were an absolute must for you (as you told me) throughout your entire life. I do understand your concerns but don't worry—nobody has yet died from vegetable-fasting for thirty days with juice, water, tea and salads. Many people deliberately go on a juice fast for a whole month annually throughout their lifetimes. It is probably one of the healthiest measures one can take to stay healthy and if struck by any illness, to get better, rather than through any other medicine. (I live solely on fruit and vegetables and never eat any of the 'substantial foods' you have been eating your entire life.) To me it is not a fast, or diet. It is life. The different direction you chose is just unfamiliar to you and to your peers. Nevertheless, if you feel that it weakens you to a point of weariness you can eat salads made of vegetables and add sea salt with lemon to it. If you are still feeling weak you may drink a little more green tea or even clear Miso soup. Vegetable soup with sea salt and as many vegetables as you like would also help your body temperature and satisfy your hunger. And most of all, rest more.

Dear Sister, as already mentioned I have been eating like that for many years and I bless every bite provided for me. I don't need to kill any creature to satisfy my hunger. Bread, butter, cake, sugar, meat, fish, processed food, candy and coffee are not good for anyone and I never eat them either. It would be a good and helpful idea to accept natural food rather than view it as a medication in times of life threatening disease. Maybe we can see it this way: Instead of thinking that cancer is due to chemotherapy, radiation and surgery deficiency, as the mainstream suggests, and that the ferocious cancer cells must be killed even if we kill the healthy cells as well; instead, understand that cancer is due to a nature connectivity deficiency. If we connect retrieve to nature and use nature's abundance to heal, then the notion is true—the produce department is our best pharmacy.

Let me know if salads and vegetable soups are helping you feel a little better and stronger. The sudden drop of processed sugars and white flour will certainly make you feel like you are withdrawing from drugs. Please understand that you are in no danger and you may lose some weight (you know that you were over the healthy weight anyway) or you may feel as if you are just surviving. But try to hold on to the strict vegetarian diet for at least a couple more weeks. The longer you hold on to it the better your body will do in regaining its self-healing powers and abilities. One of the biggest benefits your body gains of this nutritional change is ridding itself of the fungus and toxins. After all cancer is just like fungus and both hate vegetables yet crave sugar.

I think a trip to see me is not a good idea for now since you feel so weak, unless one of your sisters can help you drive since it is a pretty time consuming ride. I would rather wait until you regain some of your strength. We both know that you are a strong woman and you can do it. Many people everywhere in the world live off so much less food than even the vegetable juices and they are healthier than the meat, fish, chicken, and bread and cake consumers. Let me know how you are doing and trust in nature and goodness of the creation. It will help you on your natural journey to recuperate your natural gifts of good health.

Yours,
Yael

September 14 2007

Dear Dr. Yael,

Thank you for your last letter and for answering all my questions and easing my doubts. On the eleventh day of the fasting I am doing good considering the situation. The suggestion of the salad really makes a difference in the way I feel. I have been preparing a salad once a day from the vegetables listed by you to help me relieve some of my fear of vanishing. I am experiencing a constant pain across my waist, sometimes very sharp, especially on the left side of my body and only when I am lying down does it subside. At night I feel restless with painful cramps in my feet and legs. Overall I am surviving pretty good even though I must say that I was not prepared for the reality of this fasting diet. I am resting a lot and discontinued most of my previous activities. I only spend a few hours with my students in the classroom in the morning. Now my sisters are asking me more questions: When or how will you determine if I am cancer free? Will the lump dissolve and disappear? Or will it be by your observation? Should I get tested again? Last point, my sisters and I think you should bill me since I cannot continue to receive your precious professional care free of charge.

Please be patient with my questions, pray for me that I can continue to live this time in faith and trust in God's Will. I always keep you in my prayers with love and gratitude.

Best wishes for the coming Jewish Holidays—

Sister Paula

September 15, 2007

My Dear Sister,

Your positive email indicates your control and better attitude in dealing with your fears. The cramps are probably the body's natural reaction to the detoxification process and due to a little lack of magnesium and calcium. Now, the new nutrition regime helps to absorb the minerals and utilize them efficiently. They will not be washed out anymore as before when bonded to the sugar and sodium from your previous diet. I highly recommend applying the Pulse Electromagnetic Therapy in order to help revitalize and regenerate your vital functions. The cancer cells' status can be determined through lab tests, which I do not conduct. The lump may shrink with time and even dissolve completely but this may take a while, even when the cancer cells are dead.

Now is the time to meditate and forgive yourself, accept yourself with love and thanks for who you are and as you are. We can see the cancer cells as our most important teachers; we create them in order for them to guide us. They indicate to us how we went astray from our basic core individual with desires, beliefs and preferences and rather turned to live solely by the demands of others as well as for them—doing this in order to meet others expectations and satisfactions. It also indicates how attentive and committed we have been to exclusively meet outer demands, forgetting and disregarding our own. We basically exist in total denial of our organism, physically, mentally and spiritually and rather live just sequentially to please our surroundings as we have been raised and believed from early childhood.

Now is the time to talk to your inner-seated God and open up to yourself. Your intentions are changing thanks to a deeper understanding of your purpose on this planet in line with the responsibility you willingly assume for your health and well-being. Thus, we can do our very best for the world surrounding us without sacrificing our own interest. You are perfect because you are a human being, like any other creature on our planet earth; we are simply nature's creations and as such are each perfect in our own way. We must learn to love ourselves as you love God, because God is you and you are God. Consequently, we have to learn to respect our own life, our body and spirit, and live attentive to our inner-selves rather than in self-denial or for the benefit of only others.

This is a beautiful time of retrieving into our inner cocoon and higher spirit. At this point since you are not 'dying' any more of starvation and are rather going through this vital cleansing process, now is the time to master the mental and spiritual world. I am honored to lend you my hand in supporting you along this process and tell you that I had been on the very same course for several years. And from that point I never again eat anything that is less than pure 'cell friendly and healthy' 'cells' food,' which includes vegetables, sea weed, brown rice, millet, quinoa, fruit, beans, lentils, tofu (I make my own), seeds, sprouts (I make my own), nuts, almonds, almond cottage cheese and kefir, hemp seed, chia seeds etc. I drink green, white and red tea, charged water and water with either lemon or apple cider vinegar. I never touch any of the products I had asked you to stay away from. I never eat anything that had eyes or a mother.

I am very open and aware to the wrong thoughts I grew up with, the thoughts and principles about food I adopted very early on, and I constantly readjust to my absolute wonderful present reality and experience. I know very well how our body harbors all the old beliefs, which have a detrimental impact upon our body's health and functions. For example: The typical belief we grew up with; that we have to be good kind and pleasing to… fill in the blanks here—what were you taught? And not doing so means that we are selfish, egocentric, egoistic, inconsiderate, and careless and will be punished by God or wind up in hell, and all the many ideas alike, which is not a good place to be. We never learned the distinction between who we have to be good to or please – our peers, teachers, parents or even God. And just like you have been doing your entire life, we take these beliefs to the extreme as we literally live for the sake of our community, family, boss, children, allowing our natural drives. I too hug the 'little girl' in me and at times talk to her, share with her/me my thoughts and suggestions because I am my inner God. At times I hug her (me) to assure her (me) that we are safe, and that 'she/me/I' can do it. We all have this discrepancy between the way we understand the 'adult' person in us and the little person still residing in us albeit the passing years. Our inner spirit has no sense of time and does not care how many years elapsed since we were held in our mother's arms or laid to rest in our little crib. The main reason people need the "God concept" is so they can feel protected, guided, and unconditionally loved. As adults we cannot take these feelings for granted anymore as we 'grow up' and our parents are not around anymore to forgive and hold us, kiss and guide us. This role God takes up for us nonetheless we still need to assume responsibility for our good, security, health and knowledge from the minute our parents set us free on our path to life. At that moment we are obligated for all their duties they assumed for us as newborns. We can no longer let others decide for us what we eat, how we dress and what we must learn, because it is our duty to our own life. This is the clash amid the concept of "being in service for others" and our "responsibility for us." For, if we do not take upon ourselves that responsibility, the responsibility will take us in unpleasant painful, teaching ways, not necessarily to where we would like to go.

My brother in law's constant answer to whether he likes to eat, drink, go to sleep or to a movie has been: "I don't know. I don't care." He has been struggling with his cancer for over twenty years and declines to take any action for his recovery. In his understanding, his life is in the doctor's hands and he is not willing to assume any responsibility or do anything on his part. Do you see a doctor 'living' inside him like a tenant who takes over a rental house? He is your age and grew up by the same doctrine—be good, work hard and be responsible (for anything but yourself) so your boss will appreciate you or your school teacher will grant you high grades and those will determine whether you are good or bad. Then you may be punished if you are not good according to other's opinions. What you want is absolutely irrelevant and unimportant. His age group has not changed a thing and he too still lives by the same concepts of no connection between his conscious and training and his subconscious realm, his inner self. He never stops doing what he has to finish, even if in pain, and eats what he has been served, sleeps when it is time and meets with people who decided for him to meet. In old times, a person like him was considered as a responsible man. But now we all understand that it is wrong, harmful and instead of responsible, it is actually a very kamikaze behavior.

To listen and be in touch with our own needs and feelings is our duty given the fact that we are the one and only 'resident' in our body, mind, and being—our physical, mental, emotional and spiritual cocoon, as it is only our heart beating in our own chest and no one else's. These are only our own memories and no one else's memories. The fears are our own fears and no other's, and such are our desires. This is our life and therefore we are liable to live it and take accountability for it by becoming mindful and focused to ourselves as a whole. You light the candles in your sanctuary for the Lord you worship and the Buddhists offer their Buddha their offerings to please Him and receive His benedictions, and He never asked for your candles, prayers or their offerings. But we still go out of our way to please Him and serve Him. Why don't we understand the same rules apply for ourselves? For us being the true God of ourselves, and keep this one and only being healthy and happy.

When my father said, "Its time. Go to bed," yes it was time, but only on his watch. But was it my body's time? Was I ready to fall asleep? When your sisters 'don't believe' in nature's way to heal cancer is it based upon education or experience, or unpleasant experience with nature? Or perchance based upon "blindly following the traditional rules of discipline" only? Do they reside in your body or you in theirs? Don't your sisters realize that by not trusting nature they actually speak from both sides of their mouth? Just like you sent me the excerpt from your Bible about the trust of nature in God because he will never fail you or them, yet when it comes to the true challenge of your faith you doubt and retrieve to the instruments and chemicals that never proved to heal even one cancer patient, or even something as simple as a cold. Those who are cancer survivors survived in spite of the treatments, but most of them die and if I am wrong—why are you so scared of cancer? Are you scared of a cold or a headache as well? Do you realize how you lost your absolute trust in your Lord?

Is the food you have been served in your monastery the right and best for your health to your understanding? Or has someone else prepared it because that individual gets paid to prepare your food according to dictated budget guidelines? Is the person who prepares your meal educated and trained in nutrition and health in any way or form other than just a list of recipes? Were you ever asked what you would like to eat? Or have they ever checked whether this food is best serving your taste and health needs? You granted these individuals the trust and responsibility for your nutrition and even to plan your schedule, your vacation and time for your rest. However, your body and mind cannot accept your complete submission anymore. Your body mature and your needs have changed and so have your health needs, and as no cane or stronger glasses will help here, only radical changes in order to save your life will work, which only you can conduct.

It is time for you to look for the fruit and vegetable stand by yourself. It is time to close your office and go to sleep a good long night of sleep on time. The time has come for you to take the driver seat and the control over your life and well-being, to serve and cater to your own needs and be committed to yourself. You are over seventy-four years old now; to what age are you waiting to assume this care for yourself?

To regard that has been mentioned above you will appreciate and see this healing phase as an important pivot point in your life.

Please start now to enrich your salads with all the vegetables you like and spice with a little apple cider vinegar or fresh lemon, roast slightly seeds and nuts and

137

sprinkle them over your salad. When adding a little lemon, put in a little ground lemon skin as well as a little fresh ginger; this will not only add flavor to your salad but also serve as important healing agents with their many cardinal nutritional properties. You may also add a little extra virgin cold pressed organic olive oil and a little Himalayan salt and here you will nourish your body and mind with pure divine energy, celebrate the beauty of your colorful plate because your body does the same.

I hope that your backyard has mint and basil leaves, rosemary and Greek oregano, dill, parsley and cilantro growing to incorporate into your delicious salads. You can now eat salads made of: cucumbers, tomatoes, parsley, bell pepper, cabbage (white and red), red onions, green onions, lettuce, carrots, spinach, annis, blueberries, different seed sprouts, walnuts, pine nuts, pumpkin seeds, sunflower seeds, etc. Enjoy one or two such good rich salads daily. I know you can do it. You are on the most beautiful journey of finding the true holiness in your life—the life you were intended to embrace and enjoy by Godly order. It is nothing short of a consecrated path.

Best regards,

Yael

September 16, 2007

Dear Dr. Yael,

Today is my third week on my interesting journey to heal myself, and physically I am doing fine. I am a little tired but not as much as I felt at the beginning.

The pain I had across my waist and on the left side diminished and only occasionally comes again and the cramps disappeared as well. I lost about twelve pounds and I do not feel hungry and continue to drink the vegetable juice and enjoy the salads as you suggested.

On the spiritual and social level I am not doing so well, though my sisters continue to support me (not without doubts, questions and fears). I don't feel strong enough to rise above the subtle messages I daily receive from them.

Another friend of ours was just diagnosed with cancer, she is also a nun and is chairman of the board for Mercy Hospital, whose influence is very strong, and her surgery has been already scheduled. This is just an example of what happens around me.

My spiritual life is a struggle nobody perceives because it is so personal. I feel like a stone with no feelings and find it so difficult to pray, to meditate and to concentrate. It feels like chasing a blowing wind that never rests.

The reality of the cancer in my body also does not shock me anymore and I feel blank about it. I am possessed by challenges, yet they do not take me back to my childhood but sometimes to my younger years when I made my choices. Now that I am certainly closer to the end of my life than to the beginning, I cling to my ideals only with my will but without feelings or enthusiasm. I know that God is present in the darkness too, and I trust in His love and mercy.

The book I am reading now gives me some comfort and help. The book's title is *Free to Pray, Free to Love*, but this spiritual freedom is eluding me at the present. Please pray for me, and thank you for listening and understanding.

May God bless you and protect you always.

Love,

Sister Paula

Reflections

My biggest challenge with Sister Paula was her emphasis on the diet.

She could not comprehend the wholeness of healing herself. She couldn't find the time to come and get treatments from me, and she lived just an hour away. Sometimes the most difficult thing to see is right in front of our eyes. Furthermore, she could not appreciate the importance of rest in the healing process.

She could never conquer these challenges, but expected me or a physician to step in for her well-being. Without sleep, healthy food, joy, love, and exercise, we cannot expect life. As I mentioned numerous times along this email exchange, the difference between life and death is oxygen. When we don't eat healthy, we cannot expect our liver, kidney, and lungs to serve our body effectively. Those organs are overwhelmed by products they cannot identify as food (e.g. sugar, trans fat), and all of their energy is spent on the cleansing of toxins rather than nurturing and generating healthy blood cells, move lymphatic fluids, rush through the body to waste the processed blood, and supply fresh blood rich in oxygen and nutrients.

As we sleep, our body works hard to keep us healthy and vibrant. Sleep deprivation is toxic by itself. Human touch is also important. Never caressing a child, a man, or a woman deprives our electromagnetic functions and creates disease.

Not having real fun is just as toxic. Think of the war survivors who suffered trauma but played silly, like the Yiddish theater in the concentration camps. They survived and lived to old age because they found good laughter against all odds. Why do we hear from our ancestors that laughter is healthy? Because it stimulates the secrets of the thymus gland and the ball of health promoting hormonal functions starts to roll. Anger that stimulates the very toxic hormones secretions, but laughter stimulates the happy and relaxation hormones to pour into our blood and allow the body to relax, which promptly promotes self-healing.

I don't suggest that from this moment on we all must be silly and self-serving all the time. I hope that you see the importance in the balance we have to keep at any time and any price, between duty, fun, rest, healthy food and enjoy life. We were not born to be martyrs, in the name of god. We came to this world to make it a better place, by being better people. Good and kindness, helpful and compassion can only be achieved through the same. Being kind, compassionate, loving, and responsible for our happiness can keep us and the world around us happy and healthy.

Chapter 5: Healthy Being

Our cells are like little children. When you tell them, "You are going to die," they listen they hear and believe, especially when a teacher, a mother or father or any person in authority says the message and so they prepare to shut down and die. However, if you tell them, "You are strong, you can and will overcome the adversity and see how much fun is awaiting you," they will "get their act together" and will shift into the idea that, "Hey, look how much fun is awaiting you!"

We must always keep in mind that illness, and called disease, can never be just on the physical level of our being, or just our mind. We are a wholesome being; we are a whole galaxy in our complexity and so have to be treated as a whole. There is no medication that can heal, as long as it addresses just part of us. The same goes for mental, emotional and physical ailment.

In order to help us heal, we should observe our entire lifestyle, habits, state of mind, nutrition, social relationships, philosophy, fears, dreams and even our family life. There is no other way to truly heal, especially not cancer which is the loudest silent cry of the soul when it cannot continue to live like that anymore. It is never the breast fault, and so should never be removed.

These next conversations with Sister Paula expose the big gaps between my concept and hers.

September 20, 2007

My Dear Sister,

This is the most precious pearl I have received for a long time.

Your email reflects your beautiful healing and remission process. The physical cleansing along the meditations brings up not only physical impurity but so many deep-seated emotions surface as well. Some of them may guide you through to your suppressed anger and sadness, doubts and a re-examination of your choices, which are still steering your way though. They may not be as helpful to you anymore. Praise the Lord for your vital experience, your soul's adventure and your enlightenment. You can now see the sisters around you could most likely be in the same place as you are, encountering and probably having the same doubts and debates. Your covenant sisters have to deal with memories and disappointments as well as questionable beliefs. However, their only way to continue reaching their goal is by clinging to traditional, conventional authorized ways. Please don't expect all that much from them and simply be on guard and discriminate the right and wrong for you. They live in fear, as do all those who fear cancer or disease. Similar to most of us who don't know any better, they too chose the absolute trust in their beliefs rather than in knowledge and education. Had they been stripped off their beliefs, death would probably be considered the next best option. So naturally this is what they convey to you too.

That sister who was diagnosed with breast cancer chose the "medicine" way, which is a very deceiving method. Had she chosen differently she would have to question her very deeply rooted beliefs to which she had been clinging her entire life. This task and the extremely heavy responsibility is for most people far too frightening to deal with because it rattles and shakes their lifelong stigmas and their fundamental beliefs and concepts, as well as their convictions that the way they know is the one and only way, accompanied by the frightening idea of peeking out of their rut into the unknown. How could such a traditional oriented and schooled orthodox person possibly 'derail' from her certainties? How can anyone alike be supportive and loyal to a rebel like you?

You are a pioneer among your sisters. You dared to take charge for your own vigor and dare to raise a brow - questioning the system. You have taken a new direction and are working hard to brush some of the dusted convictions off, dared to step out of the traditional narrow minded, way overhauled authorized zone. Knowing how hard it is for you, it is clear how now you see the shift of your body as it starts to feel better and is letting go of pain and discomfort.

This is exactly my point when I say that when the body get seriously sick with a degenerative illness, it is actually at the point in which the soul is in unbearable distress, demanding and pleading for attention to the conflicts, doubts, change of concepts, disappointments, sadness, desire, wrong and harming nutrition, lack of fresh air, lack of happiness and playfulness, too much responsibility, insufficient sleep—begging for attention, insight and to be listened to. All those harmful conditions cause hormonal secretions and intoxication in our own system. Animals in nature will not be able propagate when in captivity due to their distress and possible instinctive fear and sadness. Even if they cannot explain their feelings in words, their bodies' functions will tell their story. Some wildlife actually commit suicide when in captivity because they cannot live their real healthy life. We are not different. We are nature's creatures as well. This happens the moment we start listening to our body and our being, the moment we stop consuming the toxic food, toxic news and noxious information we use in order to numb our emotions, desires and true needs, life conditions and artificial lifestyles that are not our true nature-compatible ways. As we no longer try to deaden our fears and our false beliefs with the fallaciously comforting food and illusions, and instead start to heed to our deepest and respond in a constructive way. At this point we send the message to our body saying, "no more negligence and no more suppression." now I listen and am with me/you .

This is the true implication our cells start to receive and so, of course, we get the courage, the tools and the power to fight off any disease. Our 'dialogue' with our body is just like the very soothing and empowering dialogue we would have with a person we trust. We can actually feel how our body starts to respond and function significantly better. We sense how all fear and stress lessen as we find the valor to heal and overcome all adversity that just an hour earlier put us in deep dysfunction, depression, fear and dis-ease.

You are presently enduring a tremendous hardship and struggle with the issues we discussed before your awakening from delusions. Thus, throughout these past few years, doubts in faith and real purpose started creeping up on you, as they are so hard to admit to yourself. This is part of maturing or maybe aging as well. The hardest challenge for me in getting older is the realization. Losing my illusions, the way I would see my world before through my pink glasses and having to look straight into the eyes of reality. No more daydreams and idealization of actuality, though I make my world as pretty and pleasant as I like it to be through art, craft, music, martial art, simple yet beautiful home keeping, and obviously writing.

The sister who has her mastectomy has chosen her physical solution to an inner frustration, fear, doubt, sadness, disappointment, hope, disillusions, anger, hate, cry, desperation and a very sad wake up. Do you or any of your sisters seriously believe that this surgery will cut all those suppressed emotions out? Can such a surgery truly help her heal? And if so, heal her of what? Has anyone you or I known recovered this way? Can any chemotherapy help to comfort those unresolved painful feelings?

Do you think that any surgical procedure or amputation of any part of the body can answer the unanswered prayers for a better world? Or help those victims of injustice and corruption or doubts and regret? The fear of change and the courage it takes to leave the covenant in order to start a new life or to stand up against the wrong is simply too hard and impossible for you. Were not those deep feelings the true cause for the dis-ease in the first place?

Wouldn't a better solution be the teachings of how to live a pleasant and fulfilling life in spite of the dilution? How to find joy and happiness in spite? In our daily life there is so much to be happy and grateful for even with matured adult open eyes. It is not for us to change the whole world, but the wholeness of our world. Like the water drops, each of us is one water drop that makes the ocean. You all learn to pray and thank God—do so. Thank Him for your breath and for the privilege to help the impaired.

I would like to add to this e-mail that I'm sorry about your sister and that she may have to struggle with her physical part of her (her body) but will probably never address the real cause (her soul). Just like you experienced with your knees, if we don't address the cause (our soul), the matter (our body) will break down. So you do have one week longer to go with the juicing and then maybe you will be able to start to resume 'normal' food, yet with more attendance and awareness to your inner voice. For now you are the new Sister Paula who does not numb her truth with faultily comforting toxic foods anymore. I hope that you will keep the very simple vegetarian diet for as long as you possibly can and that you will stay away from any processed food, sugar, cakes, coffee, meat, poultry, dairy, sleeplessness, anger, etc. Now you can see how the vegetarian food is not the end of the world. And anger should be tamed to manage—and stay harmless.

Please continue to pray and don't worry about the emotions that may feel even more intense and yet healthier. We must allow our emotions to surface, allow them to exist, do not hide them and do not deny them; they are part of you and they make you and us all human. Then your outlook will turn to be harmless and clear to understand and to accept allowing you to settle down in comfort or respond to whatever aggravates you. It is only natural to experience all the negative feelings. The secret to good health is not suppressing your feelings and conflicts, but rather acknowledge and address them. You will learn how vital it is to confess and even talk about that which makes you feel uncomfortable and forgive yourself. This is our nature and is the main difference between humans and the animal kingdom at large. You can see how God created our world with wisdom and miracles in your own life experience. Some of them we take for granted and some we need to learn to identify, appreciate and accept or reject. I am sure that now as you are going through your deep transformation and awakening you will return to the praying bench and to your church differently. You are not that innocent obedient young girl in an elderly lady's body any more, but a rejuvenated body with deliberate acceptance of God and His world including the good and the bad, the rich and the poor, the lucky and the less fortunate, the beautiful and the ugly. This is what the world is and since this is how God created our world it must be for a reason.

It is up to us to accept God with absolute trust and service to Him and His creation to make the difference. What other reason would God have for us to be his servants? You can now accept His rules and His laws for God has no judgment. After all we are not different than the bird in the sky, grain of sand or any flower. Just like they never doubt the reasoning behind the way they live, so should we. Please see your present condition not as a disease but more as an expression of a Dis-Ease so you can find the purpose and see your chosen path to be the right and the true one. I am very cherish you and very happy for you. Do not let anything or anyone discourage you and you will see how this journey will make you a happier, stronger, healthier and more content person than when you first started your journey. That in turn will illuminate that great light of health and vitality on your sisters, students and the people crossing your way.

I will close this email sending you a virtual hug,
Yael

September 22, 2007

Dear Dr. Yael,

Thank you for your wonderful letter; it gave me a touch of God's love, strong and reassuring. I am not going to answer now at length; I must first work on the implementation both on the physical and spiritual levels.

Thank you again for everything.

With love and prayer,
Sister Paula

September 24, 2007

Dear Dr. Yael,

I want to thank you very much for your last long beautiful letter. Yes, your words helped me greatly to face the reality of this time in my life. However, I felt that your words regarding the other sisters were a little bit too harsh. They cannot make choices they do not know about, but certainly in different times or circumstances they have been, or will be, confronted with choices to face their feelings of fear, anger, etc. The religious life that we chose and in which we are living brings us to the confrontation with the Word of God, daily; and the word of God comes through the Scripture or through other people and challenges, like for me it comes through you now as a prophet sent by God.

I would like to share with you a parable from the Gospel, the parable of the sower that Jesus told his disciples: A sower went out to sow his seeds and as he sowed the seeds some fell on the path and were trampled

158

upon, and the birds from the sky picked them up. Some of the seeds fell on the rocky ground and when they grew they withered for lack of moisture. Some seeds fell among thorns, and the thorns grew with those seeds and choked them. And some fell on good soil, and when they grew, they produced fruit a hundredfold. So his disciple asked him:

"What was the meaning of this parable?" and he explained: "The seed is the word of God. Those on the path are those who have heard, but the devil came and took away the words from their hearts that they may not believe. Those on the rocky ground are the ones who, when they heard, received the word with joy but the words have not rooted. They believed only for a short period of time and then fell away at times of temptation. As for the seeds that fell among the thorns, they were the ones who had heard, but as they went along, the anxiety and riches and pleasures of life choked them and they failed to produce fruit. But as for the seeds that fell on rich soil, they were those who, when they had heard the word, embraced them with a generous and good heart and bear fruit through perseverance."

I have read this parable many times in my life, but I had never grasped it like at the present time—the way it struck me by the deep meaning it carries and how I have been like all those different kinds of soil at different times in my life. We cannot establish in any one of those responses to the Word of God, neither the good nor the bad ones. Being on a journey also means to be alive and fearless because we are never alone, God is always with us along the way. In your letter you called me a pioneer, which made me smile. I had never been a pioneer in anything; I was always a follower and still will be a follower. I just want to follow the right way that leads to wholeness and holiness with Jesus who said: "I am the way, the truth and the life."

Today begins the fourth week of my journey and I feel good. I am not too sure about the next step of my diet. I know what food to avoid but not what food to eat to make it a sensible diet and how to figure out a daily menu from the list of foods you had mentioned in your previous letters.

So I trust your guidance and your patience with my poor experience in preparing my own food.

May God bless you always, with love and prayers—
Sister Paula

September 25, 2007

Dear Sister Paula,

Thank you for your interesting response. I enjoyed reading the wisdom in it and appreciate your modesty. The next step is not a "diet" at all. The next step is pursuing the new, and to my understanding, the better and healthier way of nutrition and quality of life. Now you can see how simple nutrition can keep us healthy and clear minded with absolute great energy, as well as wonderfully nourished. I would like to know that you start your morning with fruit. You can add to it a few almonds peeled of their brown skin, or a few pumpkin seeds, walnuts, Brazil nuts and/or sunflower seeds, chia and hemp seeds, flax seeds. Later on, have a cup of white, green or red tea. You can have a slice or two of toasted gluten, wheat, sugar and dairy free bread or rice cracker with avocado, or if you like, almond butter or, if you prefer, you can use almond, cashew, or any seed Kefir cheese.

162

The next meal should start with a big fresh vegetable salad including any vegetables you like, as long as it includes some of these: green baby spinach, green lettuce as well, kale and collard greens, beet leaves, arugula, green onions, red onion, bell pepper, tomato, cucumber, cabbage, red cabbage, carrots, green apple, walnuts, ginger root, radish, lemon and some lemon peel, and all the other good and creative ideas you can come up with. Make it colorful beautiful and rich. Please add the sprouted seeds and a little bit of organic cold pressed extra virgin olive oil, or coconut oil, apple cider vinegar or balsamic vinegar, and fresh squeezed lemon. You can choose the side dishes from the list as follows: brown rice cooked, buckwheat either sprouted or boiled. Young potato cooked in their skin. Quinoa cooked like the brown rice. Lentil seeds, preferably sprouted or cooked, kidney beans, chickpeas, peas, or any other beans you choose.

Please drink apple cider vinegar juice with water at least three times daily with or without stevia. Drink as much good water as possible. Good water can be water you will fill into a glass bottle and put on the Pulsed Electromagnetic Field Therapy Pad, which will hold the water charged for even two to three days. This is very good water for you although simply filtered water will do as well. Just like our own body the water becomes significantly better in its energy after charged, like our spirit when charged through prayers or pleasant music and a hug of love. The water we drink amazingly is influenced like we are, and changes its molecules by prayer and song, or even a smile and gratefulness. There is a reason for all religions to use water in their religious and baptizing ceremonies. Try avoiding the point in which you may get too hungry because you can always add more salad, brown rice or Quinoa, avocado, tea or fruit, or anything you feel hunger for. You can make the best combinations completely healthy. Pretty soon you may even thank the cancer to have led you to a better life on every plain of your existence.

Sending my very best regards,

Yael

September 26, 2007

Dear Dr. Yael,

Today we received your Pulsed Electromagnetic Field Therapy Device. Thank you very much. I saw the picture of it on your web site many times, but to see it closely and to touch it made me feel a little scared, but I am so happy to have it now.

Thank you for your suggestions regarding my 'new way of nutrition.' Yes, it is really very new for me when compared to the general 'normal' nutrition habits of our modern society. I have no idea what quinoa is, but I will find out. You have not mentioned some of the food I used to eat before like soymilk, soy yogurt, the veggie hamburger or other veggie preparations. Can they be part of this new way or are they not 'safe?' I may feel more confident in making splendid combinations as I go along. I want you to know that this week I feel already very good and healthy indeed. Thank you again for tolerating patiently all my questions; may God reward you abundantly with His infinite love and care. With love and prayers.

Respectfully yours

Sister Paula

September 27, 2007

Dear Sister Paula,

The most soothing words I could have prayed for are when you describe how you feel so much better. Thank you for letting me know, for it is my highest goal and biggest reward. The B3K device—the Pulse Electromagnetic Field Therapy—is going to be your health's best friend and there is absolutely no reason to be scared. All this device does is transmit energy vibrations to stimulate and enhance your metabolism, enabling your regeneration, which promotes circulation, relaxation and activates your immune system that thrives to the maximum potential for good health. (Unlike the Mastectomy, radiation and chemotherapy, which are supposed to be the means to "cure" cancer.)

You can use the big pad for the overall stimulation of all the vital functions and relaxation, twice daily on #4 for the first week and on top of it, if you have time, please use the local (small pad) on the place you are having your problem; use #2 for a start and then start to go up in numbers every two weeks. This will enhance the blood and lymphatic circulation to that area and we already talked about what cancer cells need and what makes them die off. Yes, it is better to unplug the device during thunderstorms and other times it can stay plugged in. I charge my water with the small pad by leaning the pad against the water bottle or vice versa. You can also place the water container, provided it is safely and securely closed, dry and stable, on the pad. It truly doesn't matter if you place it on the big or the small pad. As long as you keep the control box sufficiently distanced. (I would not like to have a computer in my bedroom for any price!) You can use rice milk if you like but not the processed veggie burgers, since they are made with a lot of oil, wheat and ingredients we don't want in our system. I am pleased to learn that you feel significantly better and just wait—it will get even better. The modest food like we think of as the 'poor people's' food at the end of the day is the very best food for our health. (I don't think of any McDonalds or Arby's or CFK

168

food of course.) So please stick to it. Modern food at large is very noxious.

Light and love,

Yael

September 30, 2007

Dear Dr. Yael,

Your answers guide me in all my uncertainties. Today I began to eat a little bit of brown rice and lentils with the salads but I have not yet found all the other types of foods you have suggested. It takes time since natural food is so much harder to find than junk food. I started to use the Pulse electromagnetic therapy pads, as recommended. When I first started and used it I did not feel anything with the big or the smaller pad; however, along the morning and for the rest of the day I started to feel very tired again, almost like in the first week of my fasting, as well as a little shaky, particularly in my legs and knees. I do not know why this was happening and today I am feeling significantly better, maybe because I also ate more today so I do not feel weak and shaky at all any more. I don't recall if I told you that I lost a lot of weight, fifteen pounds in this month of fasting—September. I tell you all this to let you know how

I am doing, so you can continue to direct me with your knowledge and patience.

Sometimes I feel annoyed and embarrassed by paying so much attention to my body and by the questions people ask me. The loss of weight is so evident now; I am 'swimming' in my old cloths, so much that people who know me keep asking their many questions. I offer all of this to God as my humble participations in the redemptive sufferings of Jesus, along with the darkness that surrounds me in prayer and meditations. I had the opportunity to participate in lectures and groups discussions about fragility this past week; Jesus' fragility, as well as the fragility of all humans and the people we serve, and our own. It was a good experience and I now realize how fragile and vulnerable I truly am at this point of my life, yet how it brings me closer to God, closer to the real needs of people who I serve and to the sufferings of the world at the same time. The words of the Scripture we pray every day are full of reassuring expressions that God is closer to the weak people with his strength and his Love.

"Let us give thanks to the Lord our God, who alone does great wonders and his mercy, endures forever." (Psalm 136)

I am closing now. I hope that you are well.

May God bless you always, with love and prayers—
Sister Paula

October 1, 2007

Dear Sister,

Though I have read your email a couple of days ago, I just now found a little time to reply. I apologize for that delay. Your debates and concerns about the different food options are legible. However, please let those be only your second priority on your path to recovery and health. Though the truth is that to prepare and care for your new diet requires a little more time and attention in the beginning, and that the junk food is easier to obtain, this is precisely the point. After so many years of just following and accepting everything that is served to you by others, your higher spirit and awareness require now more self-responsibility in providing for your own health and comforting needs. In the past, even though everyone knows that junk food is as it is called—junk—and is very toxic, you never raised your voice or opinion and expressed your wish to have more God's food—natural food. I recall our conversations about your nutrition and how you

173

repeatedly said to me, "This is what we get." Sometimes the healthy body has to "go on strike" to demand the proper and healthy food before a voice is heard or a change is made. The universe creates food yet men turn the food industry for an ever-growing source of revenue, disregarding their customers' and families' health damage because of their greed driven production. Some examples are fast food, anything that comes ready to microwave, or Remedia baby formula claiming to be a "wholesome nutritional formula" but contained no trace of the important vitamin B group (and in this case sadly caused the death of many babies in Israel)—the list goes on and on.

Does McDonalds care about the huge herds of cattle they raise under the most dreadful and inhumane conditions? Or the medications and suffering of those creatures let alone the people who eat these products? (The McDonalds' products, just like Dunkin Donuts and Arby's or Taco Bell, cannot even be categorized as food.) The creatures who are raised to be this 'food' and the people who eat it all get the worst modern diseases. Is this a coincidence and do the manufacturers care? No, they probably do not care because it makes them rich and the executives ride their high waves of success. Sure, they met the demands of "food on the run" but at what cost? Why do you think the cancer rate and obesity epidemic are soaring in spite of the so-called "sophisticated research" and the billions of dollars invested in those researches?

Your community serves the needy and disabled and therefore must be healthy and competent to do so, yet, if your sisters do not realize the importance of healthy nutrition going hand in hand with healthy mental and emotional conditions, how can you serve, help and maintain those who are so desperately dependent upon you? Of course it is so much easier to reach out to the unhealthy addictive foods but the price is ten folds higher to all of you. Disease and hospitals, medications and dependency, is a higher price and time consuming to pay than purchasing healthy food and preparing it for your sisters and those who eat from the same kitchen. Your sisters and brothers are falling prey to the same degenerative diseases as you have, just because they failed to maintain a proper health discipline, mentally, emotionally and nutrition wise, and succumbed to the "traditional orders", "obedience" and easy accessible junk food instead.

The other side of the coin is the simplicity that keeps mind, body and soul clear of toxins and open for purity and acceptance of divine goodness. They chose the modest and simple lifestyle and food that kept them inspired and spiritually closer to God. It is true that the food *must* be what the healthy cells thrive upon and need, and the food that can and will keep the body healthy. The healthiest people are those who eat the simplest food; they claim, "I eat to live not live to eat." So, if you eat brown rice with sea salt and variety of vegetables of all kinds, colors and forms, as well as a mixture of beans, lentils, nuts and seeds, nothing more is needed for you to heal and stay healthy. I eat the same way because it is my best liked food, because I love to stay healthy and I walk my talk. And to the most important part—please continue and cultivate the openness and connection to your inner world you discovered in yourself recently. I understand how very strange it is for you to be "so occupied" and connected to yourself, however, this is the very reason for your present health challenges. Remember how the whole church and the whole congregation gather to pray to God. And you mentioned before that it says in the scripts, "God created us in his own image." This is exactly what we have to concentrate on—the God within us, as we are responsible for our Godly life. As our body is the sanctuary of the soul, if we want a healthy soul we must keep this sanctuary of divinity in its best possible condition always, at any time, for any price and under any circumstances. There is nothing more sacred and precious than life and the only way to life is through good health and respect for oneself, physically, mentally, emotionally and spiritually.

This, my dear Sister, is the most important part in your healing expedition. Not just your food variety and not what the people around you say, think or believe, or even what your scale says or your clothes size, but the inner conviction and assurance that you are here for the sake of being alive and your responsibility for this most precious gift God has given you—your life.

Please keep it in mind and make it your first priority—starting here and now and for as long as you live.

Dear Sister, for many years I was deathly sick and since I never turn to mainstream medicine, and you know why, I had to learn on my own how to listen to what my body was trying to tell me. I had to shake off the basic ideas I was raised upon. For instance, believing that we are good only when sacrificing our own needs, wills, desires and life for the sake of others who are in need. Or for our religion or country. Yet if we look out for ourselves we will most likely be considered as bad, selfish, egocentric, egoistic, self-serving, careless, and maybe even godless.

Only when my body taught me what I needed to learn, have I stayed healthy and well. I had to learn to set boundaries, marking exactly how far I can reach out for others and when and how I had to take care of me. I must

178

admit it was not an easy task for the 'healer' in me and therefore took me quite a while to learn. Especially being a mother of three children, as one of them had special needs on top of my life long healing practice. I was well aware that I was an unwanted child to begin with. Yes, both my parents told me so since very early on that I was conceived just by accident and should not have been born—a message that followed me for many years, causing me to try my best to prove how I could be useful. I wanted to have a reason to share the planet with the rest of the world's inhabitants. I know I was not the only unwanted and abandoned child but everyone who receives that fact handles life accordingly in his or her own way. Even Van Gogh, who was so genuine in his art, was unwanted by his mother—something he suffered and struggled with his entire life.

I became an artist and a healer yet disregarded the responsibility for my own life and health. For many years I did my utmost best for others, up until my own being could not accept anymore my disregard. (As I was aging, I suddenly dropped the coin. I understood the correlation between "creature" and "creativity" and between "Creator" and "wanted" in the Hebrew alphabet.) Thus, once I healed myself from that one life threatening illness, cancer, I could not graduate from these wisdom teachings of 'Life University' and for many more years was plagued again, except this time by a very annoying skin problem. It literally forced me to alter my daily life routines, the way I dressed, and how I met people; I had to change the way I enjoyed my outdoor activities and even my rest. I could not wear any of my pants I loved and even swimming and tennis, my favored sports, had to be put on hold for over six years. Yet, I could not help myself. I could not find how and why I was creating this illness.

The illness, however, took me to the most interesting and enlightening lessons. It made me change my way of thinking and the way I handled my life. I listened to my hurting skin and knew that there was important information my body was trying to convey to me from my inner soul and emotions. I had to learn to obey my own body dictations by close attention to my own concerns, desires, resentments and needs, and to make major changes and very different choices. Like, for instance, getting rid of old life philosophies and myths that did not work for me anymore. I had to stand ground and express what I felt here and now and not procrastinate my feelings in the effort to "be good" and considerate of others—solely. I had to learn to navigate my life in a wiser way between my feelings and of those surrounding me. I had to learn a brand new language in order not hurt others as I was setting my boundaries in a crystal clear way, unlike before, and being responsible and attentive to myself.

Thus it sounds so trivial that when we feel thirsty but do not get up to take a cup of water because we have to "be good" at work or we cannot go to the bathroom because it is "not nice" to do so while at a meeting or in class. Or if we feel uncomfortable when working to stop our spouse from talking to us, disrespecting our need to concentrate and let him simply wait until we lift our eyes. Not everyone can say, "Please let me finish, I am very busy now." Or, when you know that the person in front of you, be it your child, your spouse or your friend, is telling you a lie and you don't say right there, "Try again. It doesn't sound true." Or when you are a guest in someone else's home and you are very thirsty, yet feel embarrassed to ask for a glass of water but no water is offered so you stay thirsty rather than ask. Or when you are very tired and have to attend a meeting or a prayer, or you have to stay at your friend's party or have guests instead of taking a break and rest, you literally force your body and mind to do all those things against your needs only for the sake of being good, polite, minding your manners, etc. Those are just small and trivial examples I am bringing up in order to elaborate about the very basic and natural needs we learned to hide and tuck in for the sake of being regarded as adequate, conformist, well-mannered and well-cultivated, socially well-behaved, and in order to please our social environment by meeting their expectations of us.

Nonetheless, throughout the years we turn those little incidents into our second nature and completely disregard or listen to these necessities. It happens a lot in congregations like your covenant, between husbands and wives, between soldiers and their commanders, and at work and schools.

We are raised and trained to accept all the expectations, society regards as well behaving yet disregarding our own vital functions and needs, suppressing and procrastinating them, and we develop these conditioned reflexes, anxieties, peer pressure responses, or even tuck our true emotions in when we need to put up a facade.

When we fear or when we are sad and anxious, we even apologize for the feelings we feel and try to suppress them with medications, unless we pass out before; like with depression, anger management, restlessness, concentration difficulties, and sleeplessness and more.

Every ailment or disorder is a reflection of our inner world, a new step in our evolution and growth, yet, if we don't respond and don't open up to the message our body tries to convey, we cannot heal.

Why do you think has the meditation practice been proven to help reduce high blood pressure, high cholesterol and help sleeplessness, and combat depression better than any known medication? Think of it this way: When you were four years old the clothes and shoes you could wear at the age of two did not fit you anymore. Then when you were fourteen years old the same happened with the cloths you could enjoy at the age of four. They again simply did not fit your body anymore and you had to change your garments and shoes as you grew up and changed and had to let go of your favored clothing of early childhood. Would you think that the same thoughts you had at the age of ten could still serve you at the age of eighteen?

The same goes for our emotional, mental and spiritual growth. We outgrow our old thinking habits, myths and patterns, our old fears and joys, and have to adapt to new ways of understanding our surrounding world, whether it is through learning and education or through our life experience and maturing. We have to adjust to the diverse and new events and comprehensions.

Unfortunately, some of us cannot bare it, and even fear the change to the point that we decline transformation and continue to adhere to the old ways.

However, life goes on and we are uncovering new understandings as the learning never ends until we die.

Not just our clothing size needs to be adjusted and changed in accordance, but our decision making, our belief system, our perceptions, our trust and values, our likes and dislikes and faith. Though not easy at all, especially for the clingers to the known and traditional and for the kind of people who can't help but be rigid, fearing the next step in life—this process is called of change, however, is *called* Life. Those who get seriously ill are the ones who cannot endure the change.

It creates a deep friction and conflict in us so much that we may even lose our health for.

Many men start to lose ground in their life once they retire unless they have a good plan and are prepared for that stage in their life, as they feel "useless" or "good for nothing anymore." This is just like women whose children grew up and left their nest. If those women don't prepare to face that stage in a very creative and assertive way, they will most likely join the many millions alike who visit their doctors frequently for depression, sleep disorders, arthritis, cancer and other "Empty-nest" symptoms—and these patients are numbed with medications, not treated. How much better would it be if their doctors guided them through this transition rather than suppressed it with pills? The true name of diseases like these is—change.

We have to grow and embrace the way our life alters, accepting the fact that nothing in life is so stable and sure like the changes. If we try to swim against the stream and fight the trend, we jeopardize our well-being. Go with the flow; that is the way the universe works. Taking care of oneself means taking responsibility. Who should be liable for us as adults if not ourselves? It is even harder to conceive for a nun, I know.

Only if we reach all the way inside our mind, soul, spirit, behavior-patterns and social conditions and habits we adopted, can we find the true way to solve our health problems and resume good health in a strong body mind and spirit.

Best wishes,

Yael

October 3, 2007

Dear Sister,

Did you watch the news today? They removed a woman's breast because of wrong diagnosis. The statistics: 10% of diagnoses are wrong. Keep your body as God created it for you.

Be well,

Yael

October 5, 2007

My Dearest Sister,

Some times I wish I could just sit with you for a whole month and just write your story. I wanted so much to become a nun (Jewish nun? funny!) and now I have the privilege to treat a nun. I wish I could be an author of a book about the differences between women's lives as nuns and women from all different life paths. Wow! Just thinking about it makes my hands tingle. I smile whenever I think about it. Though English is neither yours nor my mother tongue, you still do very well writing your email to me. You do express yourself very well in spite of your self-doubting. Which kind of differences you refer to is unclear to me, but yes I know they are there. The biggest one between you and I is the submission to religious, orders and tradition; you accomplished being a conformist and I am always questioning and challenging, since I am a nonconformist, which is my nature. I am sending you my very best wishes on your birthday and pray that we will

189

meet on this earth many more years and will learn by sharing many more important lessons as we have been since we first met. In any case, you are my closest encounter of everything I have learned about living for the sake of service of the divine, and it is a very interesting learning experience for me.

Yours,

Yael

October 8, 2007

Dear Dr. Yael,

I received your short email from October 3rd about the news and yes I did watch the news that night and wondered if my diagnosis was included in that wrong 10%. But how can I know? I also received your long letter dated October 1st, which gave me a lot of "food for thought." Every time you open a little window into your life I am always amazed. I admire your great spiritual insight. It is interesting to watch how suffering made you such a tower of strength, a beacon of light and a prophet for our confused modern world. I told you how I always was a follower and believe that God protected me in such ways I could never understand or question. At this point as I am in the process of self-searching and I do not see the need to change my beliefs and my commitments to the Church, to my Institute, and especially to my vows. There is one thing I can clearly regard as necessary to do and I am working at it. I must revitalize and deepen my commitments.

As I recall our last conversations, I shared with you the danger in religious life when even the most sacred moments become routine and the vice of complacency or self-righteousness creeps in and destroys any chance of really getting close to God in spirit and truth. I am concentrating on this effort at this moment with the help of the Holy Scriptures, a lot of prayer, trusting in God's mercy and letting go of worries, plans or goals to achieve on the professional, or any other, level. However, in order to establish a true connection between this spiritual effort and the simplification of the food is a difficult task for me. The simple food I eat as I follow your guidance is not simple at all. When I was still living at home in Italy in the 40's we lived in a small village out in the country. We were very poor and lived off the vegetable garden in our backyard. The food was really very simple and crude. It was throughout the time of the Second World War and was our only means of surviving. Now I have to drive miles to find that simple and fresh food, further even than to come and see you, though traveling in the opposite direction. I have to go to the upper class neighborhood in order to find these fresh fruits and vegetables, which are so much more expensive than the non-organic on top of all that. Some of your nutrition suggestions I cannot not find yet, like for example the wheat and gluten free bread. You said that this has been your nutrition for so many years already; yet, I cannot see it possible for me. I hope for the moment when I will be free of cancer and when I will be able to resume my regular food – the common food. When we talked about diet it never crossed my mind that organic food even existed, but you may have assumed that I knew. I first learned about it through your list of suggestions when you wrote, "the vegetables must be organic." So please forgive my ignorance. My group of people is supporting me in every way possible and I will continue with the organic food as long as I have to. I energize the water and hopefully it will help my cells, although I do not feel anything while using it.

Thank for your patience on this long letter. May God bless you and always protect and reward you with the abundance of His love.

With love and prayers,

Sister Paula

October 10, 2007

My dear Sister,

This is the dissimilarity between the common medicine approach and the approach of natural health. In the natural health method we learn to become aware of the life habits that lead to sickness and by gradually changing those old customs we keep both the changes and our good health continues as we consistently keep our new and improved way of life permanently; the conservative medicine approach labors to remove the symptoms and only rarely suggests the option of a fundamental change of life habits. Like for example: Mainstream medicine does not ask us to change our diet, exercise, play, heal our 'victimhood' or 'martyr-hood' or control issues, power and anger management issues, and rather suggests we put our physical and/or emotional needs at the very end of our priority list. When we feel we do not deserve to address our necessities and problems first and as soon as possible, assuming it is appropriate to wait until we have been taking care of

195

everyone else. Think about rape victims who never spoke out, including domestic rape among married couples, abuse, trauma, shock, anxiety, and so much more. Many people like you live under such selfless conditions because this was their choice at a very young age and they had never entertained the possibility of self-care, pleasure, sexuality, or attempted to satisfy their own personal desires and needs. To "resume the old ways" is no different from the compulsive smoker or substance abuser that stops smoking yet cannot wait to get back to his old habits and addictions. (Selflessness as a way of life to the point of self-denial and self-damage and is in my opinion, an addiction as well.) And the damage is doubled when resuming "the old way." When the body or the psyche experience and learn to avoid the harmful agents, the sensitivity to the harmful properties becomes tenfold higher than it was before the person experienced the healing process. This is how the organism builds caution against those harming agents and develops the self-protection mechanisms. Whether the trauma experienced was due to emotional negligence or any other abuse, or even social or nutritional negligence; this self-conservation system saves us from continuous damage that we just cleared off.

This is another vital part of our immune system and is our "health and life preservation" and our "inner guard" instinctive system as well. Therefore, when resuming the "old" patterns we break and shed our trust in our own promise to our own life force and actually break the immune system's wall and the body breaks down even worse than it had before. Take for example a person who stopped smoking after thirty years of smoking. That person, after overcoming the withdrawal crisis, will soon develop a clear intolerance to cigarette smoke when others smoke in his presence. This happens when the body received permission to protect itself and knows by now that this odor, smoke or taste is a life-threatening product. Like anxiety, or resentment to the point that the individual will feel the drive to get up and leave the room, or watery eyes, cough, anger, nausea, or he may even approach the smoker and demand his own right for clean air. This is how strong the body responds to its own life preservation instincts after weaning off a harmful addiction. Now if that same person would resume the smoking habit the damage would get significantly worse than it had been before because the receptors will be removed and it would be "caught off guard" in a pictorial description and the body's reaction will be of an "unarmed soldier" who receives the devastating and dangerous bullets yet has given away his weapon to resist it anymore.

Can you please now look and see your priority list clear and bright and see that your place on your responsibility and priority list is at the very bottom of your list? Remember that you are seventy-four years old and lived by the "common diet" and followed a nun's life style since you were just eighteen years old. Now you are just a few weeks into these major and drastic changes in your life on the mission to save your life. It may take a while before you feel the results and before you may reap the fruits of your new way you so eagerly expect. Even as a nun you should realize that health, regardless how much we invest in it monetarily, as well as the time and effort, is after all our most important and most precious asset which we can never stop investing in and never stop cultivating and let off guard. You, as a nun eventually will cost your community significantly less money when you treat yourself the natural way than had you been treated the general way. Please try to learn how not to feel guilty if after so many years of committed service there comes a time when you need to take care of yourself as well. It is your born right and it is your duty, as well as the privilege of all the people who have been working with you all those years to help you resume good health.

Everyone deserves to be healthy. We all deserve good health and the support of our families or community on our path to regain our lost and compromised well-being. This is the highest priority—It is your duty to get well no matter what the cost may be.

In regards to the pulse electromagnetic field therapy, I would continue the same numbers and each week go up one number until you reach the last number at which point, you can start to simply alternate.

Have a beautiful weekend.

Truly yours,

Yael

October 12, 2007

Dear Dr. Yael,

Thank you for your reply and there is no need to apologize for the delay. I understand that you have many important things to do for many more people. I also want to clarify my concern about the food by saying I did not mean to go back to my old nutrition patterns prior to the cancer diagnosis. The nutrition I had in mind is the same you outlined in the link *Introduction to the Simple Way to Good Health*, which is very similar to what I am doing now with the exception of the organic food. From your reply however I realize that I may be wrong in thinking that the organic food can be discontinued safely at a certain point. I am determined to continue this natural way to good health on every level that is required, nutritional and spiritual, even if it is difficult, especially with the lack of acceptance and belief by our society at large. You certainly know this better than I do. I am certain that perseverance can make the whole experience easier and I thank you for your advice.

Another issue I would like to ask your advice: How should I handle social events when I have to travel or participate at retreats or conventions, which of course, require dining away from home. Sometimes I can take my food and at times I can just sit with the others and have just water if it is for just a short lunch or dinner. But when it is for more than one day I do not know what I should eat. I could always have a salad, but would it matter if it would not be organic? I am really concerned about all the adjustments. All those events are coming up in November and December, which I have to attend as well as a friend's funeral; he died of leukemia and was exactly my age. I do not know much about his life and nutrition because he was in Australia and returned home to die. He was the bishop who represented our church there. Those events make me feel even more thankful to God for guiding me to you and for the good health that He is already giving me now.

Just as I intended to inquire about your book I was happy to find your email tonight that announces the imminent distribution of *Giggling Dr. Green* to the public. Congratulations! Now I am forwarding your email to my sisters and to as many people as I can knowing it will be just like a little drop in the ocean but I hope to make at least some people question and doubt the conventional medicine and the use of medications.

May God Bless You always with love and prayers—
Sister Paula

October 13, 2007

Dear Sister Paula

As you probably know by now my nutrition suggestions are not just what I preach but what I keep and do and have done for the past thirty years, and although I certainly run into some difficulties at social events, it is still feasible and easy to handle.

From the Asian culture I learned about their dried food and how very convenient they are in such events. For example, mung bean noodles, sweet potato noodles, seaweed and miso soup, as well as dried mushrooms, are all very easy to prepare. Just stir for a short time in hot water and they will be good food for you within just a few minutes. On trips I take dried mushrooms and dried seaweed, dried vegetables, soy nuts, and all that needs no refrigeration. I have always walnuts, almonds, chia seeds, sesame seeds, pumpkin seeds, hemp seeds, dates, sunflower seeds, brazil nuts with me and don't require any preparations and are the best source of nutrition one can ask for. The dried food needs just a little bit of seasoning, like apple cider vinegar or red wine vinegar and fermented coconut sauce, and you can prepare a better tasting and more nutritious meal than all the processed food served at those events. Tofu can be purchased in airtight packaging that needs no refrigeration either in every grocery store and is very simple to prepare as well as miso, which is fermented soybeans paste and will make the best soup with just hot water like you would prepare instant coffee. Miso has many more health promoting properties as probiotic and good healthy proteins that make it well worth keeping in our "healthy food" collection anyway. For dessert a little bit of dried, unsweetened or fresh fruit and nuts or almonds will serve you deliciously as well. Brown rice cakes are very easy to obtain and serve you well on trips and events with dates or nuts or any fruit. All those ingredients are light in weight, convenient to store and carry around, they are good for your health (and when you eat any of them you can never get an upset stomach) and you can eat as much as you like. Here in the US you can find salad bars and freshly packed green leaves salads and even cut fruit bowls in every supermarket you go. Be a little creative in preparing your meals. I mentioned the fresh fruit, vegetables, nuts and seeds you can find everywhere and could probably be served even in most of your social events. Though they may not be organic, they are at least not processed food or salt and chemicals loaded with artificial colors and flavors or any preservatives. All those food ingredients are not machine made foods that have a longer shelf life than anyone of us. Most food that is served in social events should never even be regarded as food in the first place and if you stay away from it you already gained a significant chunk of healthy advantage. See how in every organic or natural food we need to insert dry bay leaves or refrigerate it in order to prevent pests from spoiling it, versus the artificial food even pest and worms don't like to touch and eat. Just like no pest or worm would ever try to eat concrete or lime, yet the commercial grown cows feed off it for faster weight gain and lower expenses, and people actually eat the meat derived off

206

those poor abused animals and call it substantial food. (It is true—concrete makes it substantial).

When you get a chance take a look at other people's luggage you can see what people put in their suitcases wherever they travel, like big bags of medications, inhalers and oxygen canisters, enemas, special back supports and extra pillows, creams and lotions, blood pressure and blood sugar gages, extra jewelry and special event shoes, etc. I don't need to pack all of those and so I have plenty of room left for the dried food bags together with a bag filled with a mix of lentils, chickpeas, mung beans, and maybe even fenugreek seeds and buckwheat. It takes just five minutes when I arrive at the retreat; all I need to do is soak a teaspoon full of the seeds and rinse them twice daily with water. Within just a few hours I already have my little organic vegetable garden sprouting for my delicious healthy meal. You can eat them just the way they are without any preparations or cooking or add them to your miso soup with seaweed and lightly cook them with the soaked dried mushrooms. All that could be a little "food for thought," "humongous food for your body" and for you to realize how easy it is for us even when we are on trips. At social events of just lunch or dinner I don't have to drink just water and see how others enjoy their feast. I can take with me a dried fruit bar, a few cashew nuts or walnuts, dates and dried fruit of any kind I like, a bag of white or green or maybe even fruit tea in my little briefcase, just like others would take their medications, makeup or cigarettes and lighter with them, and enjoy celebration with all the rest.

Another little idea which may change your feeling on such occasions: I feel so blessed to have all those options and feel for all of those who have to share the artificial foods and their sad and harmful results, which usually will sound later on like, "I wish I had not eaten that creamy cake or ice cream, I feel so bad now." Or, "Every time I am on these retreats I return home sick for a week or two before my body gets rid of all the food they serve." Or, "It takes us forever to lose the weight we gained from the food we have when we are away." Yes, we may pay a little extra, but not much. And always keep in mind how much more expensive and time-consuming illness and inhibiting and limiting pain, can cost a lot more.

Another nice way to eat well and inexpensively (not on trips of course) is to consider the option of growing your own leafy vegetables, tomatoes, cucumbers, and even peppers in your backyard or even in pots. It is inexpensive, easy to cultivate, fresh, healthy and delicious to eat. Imagine how tasty and mouth watering a vegetable can become when grown in your own yard with your love and care. This energy alone makes every food we eat tenfold tastier and significantly richer in its health service than anything we purchase. The fertilizer can be made of kitchen scrapings you can compost.

I am so repelled by those greedy reckless pharmaceutical and medical terrorists.

Thank you for your wishes and prayers and most of all for your trust.

Love,

Yael

October 13, 2007

Dear Sister,

I enjoyed our last conversation. Since you feel that you have lost too much of your weight I suggest that you leave the very strict diet now so you won't disappear and start to add more vegetable proteins to your diet. It can be any vegetable protein you choose. There is no vegetable that does not contain proteins and if you stick to a nice variety of fruit and vegetables, brown rice and almonds, maybe you will get all the protein you need. Green peas, fermented soy products like tofu, tempeh, almonds, all seeds and nuts (best raw though lightly roasted are good and delicious too) and all sprouts (raw) have plenty of protein. Beans, mung beans, chickpeas, and lentils are all protein rich foods.

From our correspondence I can see how you are getting so much better. Not all lumps disappear as some stay and become inactive as far as cancer cells activity, and as long as they are not harmful and do not threaten your

210

health anymore, when they die off and become sedentary, you are fine. They "serve" us as a little memorandum to remind us of our important teachings in mastering our healthy balance. I would like to reveal a little secret to you. For many years I have had a black mole on my right leg, which according to many physicians (I knew at my dancing group) should be checked and removed, since it was for sure carcinoma. You know they were right, yet I never believed in the doctor's approach to cancer and instead found it useless to have it checked. After all, we all knew what it was. I knew the reasons that lead me to create that cancer—it was all the extremely difficult years I went through during my time on the Jordanian borders fearing the night and day infiltrations of terrorists in order to kill and capture women and children. The father of my children, who was never around and when he was would be very abusive to them, was always out for other women and this also contributed. My family never cared about my children or I and so naturally never supported us. As for my in-laws, my complexion was "too dark" for my father-in-law (I am dark olive) and so I could not be accepted into the family and deserved no support at times of adversity, like for example right after the war, or when their son would just take off and ignore his children. The worries about my children's and my own very basic needs—whether or not would I find a way to feed us. Plus the Chron's I was born with, my dairy and gluten intolerance, and the immigration to this wonderful new but challenging country alone with no help or support with my three children—all this contributed to the mole to change into cancer. For all those years I was gluten and lactose intolerant yet unaware of it, I had heavily bloody stools, and since I refused to accept any medications and insisted on finding the reason for those profuse and dangerous hemorrhages. In spite all my knowledge; I could not uncover the reason for my body's illness. Not knowing why I could not absorb and utilize any minerals, vitamins, proteins and instead lost more of my vitality by the day. I was very sick with absolutely no help or support, with close to no hope as well. I had ulcerated intestines for many years and when I had an attack I would bleed like a faucet. As I mentioned a few times already, I was not aware of the dairy and gluten intolerance I had since early childhood and in very stressful times the ulcers in my intestines would bleed profusely. Not even my mentor and great teacher of natural health and classic homeopathy could help me. He suggested that I resort to antibiotics and steroids and warned me that if I would not use them I would soon die. But I refused. I had seen my aunt deteriorate and run down on all of those drugs and it was absolutely not an option for me. Since my early childhood the food I had was based on bread and cheese, if I had any food at all. My father never believed in any diets and all I received were just penicillin shots for my frequently recurring inflammations that never stopped. Then my body broke down and this mole started to grow and became very ugly. Thanks to that mole I learned how to listen to my body and emotions and I changed my attitude and started to better 'communicate' with my emotions. And so, when I got angry, disappointed, worried, upset and hurt, I dealt with my pain and did not hold it in anymore. I have learned to deal with problems and difficulties in my life I could control and let go of those I had to leave to the universe to control.

I replaced fears with more trust in the goodness and kindness, of myself, to myself and of the universe, and found so much more peace in just acceptance and gratefulness. I did not fear death but just took my life one day at a time, more aware, better at standing up for myself and when needed, I started to speak out rather than keep quiet, harboring my words in a hurting heart. I suddenly learned how my past and my childhood led me to interact with people in a very self-harming way, which I hated. I hated my need to be accepted and do my utmost to satisfy that need. I would go out of my way to please the world surrounding me. It took me a while before I finally grasped that I cannot make the whole world accept and love me and that I should better accept myself and love myself as the universe loves me. In that shift in perspective I found acceptance from the surrounding world and I could finally live in peace with myself. I could finally accept the fact that my childhood was during one of the worst wars the world had ever experienced in history. I grew up surrounded by so much objective fear, hunger, shock, grief, sadness, hate and hopelessness and all that horror understandably left its marks globally, on the whole world, as it has on my close family and me. I finally realized how it was time to go on with my life, be the creator of my own happiness, do my very best for the world I came in touch with, and let go of the past and its imprints upon my view of life, love and acceptance. Unlike before when I would get upset and very worried about those who chose death rather than modify their nutrition and lifestyle, I continued to treat people all those years, yet had stopped 'playing God' and left the final choices to them and the universe. I just did my very best. I also stopped feeling trapped and set myself free by changing the conditions and circumstances that I needed to change – all of the circumstances that made me feel enmeshed. If my reality and life conditions could not be changed I successfully changed my state of mind and accepted what could not be changed and simply stood up for myself, found all that was enjoyable and be grateful for and adjusted my core beliefs.

From then on, I clearly stated my boundaries and where they had been trespassed I "repaired my hedges". I have cherished every food crumb I've eaten since then and learned to sooth, yet disregard, the fear of lack and the fear of existence. I changed to be a happier person and realized how every one of us was born to do the best we could on our planet and one day we all will have to say goodbye to matter and evolve into the godly energy. I have been enjoying the healthy cells nutrition and declined any tempting dish. I never touch any man-made foods that have been carefully engineered only to allure us by the junk food industry. After all, if we were created in His image we should eat only the food we would have served a newborn (I don't regard any processed baby food as food either). Though I never ate fast of junk food and since I had never seen McDonald's burgers grow on a bush or tree, nor French fries being reaped in the fields, I wouldn't eat them. I had never seen a river run of Coke, or an ice cream field.

I had been using the Pulsed Electromagnetic therapy device too and was one hundred percent positive that I was rebuilding and regenerating my health and my immune system, which I have. And you know what? I had to learn to respond differently to many challenges in my life and change my attitude.

I am so happy now but the most important teacher and trigger in my life and health was this black spot on my leg. It is my 'self healing gage' that is there to refresh my awareness to what I feel and help me navigate my life. It is my indicator and signal light for the right balance of my nutrition and respect to my health and life. You know it looks a little funny now because the deep dark color started to recede and change as healthy skin is growing from within. Yes, my dear Sister, you are older than me and in spite of all the drama and fear around the word cancer, I simply don't worry. Zen monks say, "The sad part in death is not the fact that the person dies but the fact that he did not live." This is exactly how I live, by simply living and seeing the brightness, the beauty and the happiness of our universe and like a little candle, I try to illuminate as much light as I possibly can in this universe. I am very happy each day so that when I die I can be happy and grateful for the days, hours and years I have had.

Now eighteen years later this brown spot on my leg makes me smile every time I see it because it helped me look deeper into myself and made me aware and gave me the ability to change myself from deep inside for the better. Would it be wiser to cut it out and be fed with chemotherapy and radiations? Would I still be here to write you this letter? I truly doubt it, but the healthy skin completely hushed the black cancer cells away and my health is excellent. One of my friends a nurse who worked in the cancer department in Canada said to me one day, "Are you aware of the big black spot on your leg?" I smiled and said, "Sure." And she said, "It doesn't look good at all." I said, "Yes, I know, it is angry." She said, "Yes, it looks very angry." I said, "It hates my chemotherapy and it was just given a mega portion of it."

"So," she added, "Do you receive chemo?" I answered, "Yes." "In the oncology department?" she asked. "Sure," I said, "My oncology department." She blushed of confusion and asked, "Your oncology? How?" "Well," I said, "cancer cells hate raw lemon, and you can really drive them crazy when you add propolis solution to it, and it's even worse when they are served baking soda for dessert. This is how I have been treating them. Now, a few days after that lovely meal they get red and mad. But isn't the best sign of active auto immune system redness, heat, itch and swelling?" I asked.

Now she looked at it a little closer and said, "Your healthy skin is pushing the bad cells out and it is healing beautifully." I said with a huge grin "You forgot that I am a natural born fighter and so are my healthy cells. Here see, we won the battle." She turned silent and didn't add a word.

And for you, please know even if you can still feel your lump you may consider it as your best friend. It guided you, and still does, to improve the care and consciousness of your body and soul.

The lump opened your eyes and led you to take better care of your health and awakened your immune system, which was in severe jeopardy. It was your very last call for a major change or else your body would probably collapse and resign. Thanks to this lump you have made those radical changes and have learned so much about health, nutrition, attitude, yourself, even learned to listen to your feelings and needs, things you had never dared to attend to before you were diagnosed and even lived with the notion that those are sinful. As weird as it may sound, the lump has been your lifesaver. This lump you dreaded so much led you to allow yourself to tell your sisters what you need and even let them know how much life meant to you. So, just continue to stride on your journey until you find this little friend, your precious lump, is simply there and like the shadow that scared us when we were little children, disappearing when our mother turned on the light.

Do you recall the research I talked about when it became clear how healthy cells have little glimpses of light, versus cancer cells that have none? It makes so much sense, because healthy cells thrive when oxygen is absorbed, and cancer cells die off it. Oxygen is like fire, light and green. All green leafy vegetables are green thanks to the photosynthesis they metabolize with light, which is what we receive when we eat them. Photosynthesis comes from the light, and the green helps the body to create hemoglobin, which is the oxygen transmitter in our healthy system. Dead food will never be able to enrich our body with oxygen. So, here you see the correlation between light, oxygen, healthy cells and the darkness of the cancer cells—simply put—enlightenment heals.

Do not worry, look at it as your greatest teacher who 'forced' you to change your lifestyle to get rid of the toxic foods and angers and cherish life.

Love,

Yael

November 9 2007

Dear Dr. Yael,

I am excited about your new book *Giggling Dr. Green.* I wish to see that book in every home and every household. It sure will save many lives and prevent lots of suffering and grief. This I know for sure. Did you see the news last Saturday night? I thought about you when I saw those parents who were threatened with incarceration because of their refusal to vaccinate their children. I tried to picture your reaction to all that and to the old doctor's comments. Even I felt furious with just the little knowledge I have in this matter.

I am continuing my healing process well and feel fine with good physical energy, peace of mind and am letting go of worries about things I cannot change. Last Tuesday I lost my old dog and felt very sad but I had to let her go, for she was very old. I thank God for all the years I enjoyed having that beautiful friend. I continue my new nutritional lifestyle very faithfully and apply the pulse electromagnetic field therapy three times daily, once with the whole body mat and twice more using the intensive applicator. I used #4 for the most, yet sometimes #7 when my time allows, and I rest because it still makes me feel shaky. I hope that I have been using it properly and the results will be in accordance. I used the intensive applicator on the lump, which is still there though it has changed somewhat. Sometimes I feel a mild pain or a sense of pulling in that area, which I hope is a good sign. My only health complaint for now is a swelling of the left ankle and leg, which persists in spite of my effort in natural ways like hot and humid applications, elevation, etc. I will be grateful for any suggestions you may have. I hope that you will find a little time to write me in spite of your busy life. I like to wish a very Happy Thanksgiving to you and your family.

May God Bless you always with the abundance of His Love, with peace and success in all your activities.

In prayers love and gratitude,
Sister Paula

December 6, 2007

Dear Dr. Yael

Thank you very much for your newsletter. I really appreciate your many helpful suggestions for better health, including your book suggestions.

However, the most exciting news was that your book was finally born. I congratulate you again for your wonderful accomplishment and will start reading it and recommend it to others as much as I can. I was very busy these past few weeks and did not find much time to write, but I did not let the extra activities disturb my inner peace. This is a special time of the year, the holiday season, and as you guessed luckily the whirlwind of shopping and parties do not affect me at all. I feel fortunate to avoid all that. In our Catholic tradition the four weeks before Christmas are called the "Season of Advent," which is an ancient Latin word meaning, "coming." As we wait for the Savior to come, remembering through the Scripture, the Prophets, the long waiting of the Old Testament until Jesus was born.

It is a time for more prayer, for penance and for extra efforts to help those in need. The Season of Advent is the perfect opportunity to continue my new way of nutrition, which I have been doing anyways. I am healthy and strong. I use the B3K daily. I am grateful for all the good fortune in my life and very grateful to you for guiding me the right way.

I hope you are also doing well and that God is watching over you and your activities and family, abundantly. I am closing with the words of an ancient Advent hymn: "O come, O come, Emmanuel, and ransom captive Israel, That mourns in lonely exile here, until the Son of God will appear, Rejoice! Rejoice! O Israel! To thee shall come Emmanuel." In our Christian Bible the name Israel indicates our soul in need of redemption. May this wonderful season fill your heart with light and joy. Happy Hanukkah!

With love and prayer,

Sister Paula

Reflections

Sister Paula realized how her entire life she had followed a concept she thought was the one and only absolute truth in the world. Then her sacred walls started to crack around her yet she still held fast to her cracking walls in forgiveness and disbelief.

At that point all came together as her inner "walls" which were her own physical health came tumbling down as well, and worst of all her belief system that started to shake violently.

Sister Paula had to start thinking for her own and assume responsibility for her health and life, yet not out of her liberate educated and intelligent choice, but out of fear for her life.

The difference she could endure was just clinging to me as her healing avenue rather to her fellow nuns or the doctors. The sad part was that she was so tunnel-visioned that she could not see farther than her juicing machine, which she used instead of medications.

The concept of "I am valued by my service" and that life was secondary on her priority list got in her way in her healing process. Juicing made sense to her, it could be compared to swallowing a medication, yet, rest, relaxation, emotional healing, love, natures rights for happiness, were too foreign for her, and so she walked just part of the natural healing path.

I mentioned to her how balance was the most important part in good balanced health, but I was wrong to believe that such an extreme religious fanatic person would be able to comprehend that vital point for a healthy life.

The fear of healing our own body without clinging to something or someone was simply unbearable for Sister Paula because it demanded her to mature, become independent, and take responsibility for her own well-being. For many of us taking control at work, our family, children or spouse, or running a huge company is less frightening and easier to handle than taking the same control and responsibility for ourselves. It never really materialized with my friend Sister Paula and therefor she repeatedly bagged me not to abandon her, as she would pray to Jesus.

The concepts of healing, help, responsibility, trusting, safety, and the whole idea around maturing and becoming strong and self reliant, was to her like to so many who can relate to her—an equivalent to drowning in a pond, with no lifeguard available. The notion of "I need support," rather than, I am strong, trust myself, I can learn how to provide my own needs is foreign not only to sister Paula but to a significant part of our human society.

However, not controlling our own well-being, health and life and leave it to others is just like letting others eat for us, digest for us, learn for us and sleep for us. We are the only entity residing inside our life, and so the only ones who are solely responsible for this life.

Chapter 6: Bittersweet Success

I never stopped believing in Sister Paula. As I watched her struggle to regain her health, I was amazed that her successes did not inspire her to make the adjustments needed to keep her hard earned health. I was concerned because if she slipped into the same lifestyle that made her sick in the first place, she would most likely get sick again.

She continued to leave everything in God's hands. It is a great thing to have faith, but it's very destructive to use faith as an excuse to hold onto unhealthy choices. Our healthy choices should enrich our faith, and if our faith encourages us to abuse our bodies, then it's not very useful.

Our health demands a commitment from every part of our life—not just our diet and using natural medicines. As I received these emails, I wondered of Sister Paula would always be distracted by the little things and never put the entire program to work so she could enjoy lasting health.

December 8, 2007

Dear Sister Paula,

Thank you so much for all this good energy sent my way, as it is shining from your email. I am happy to find how much stronger and healthier you are getting. You do not need to thank me just the universe, yourself and God, because I was just sent your way and had been given the tools to help you as many others before (and hopefully after you as well) for as long as I am here.

So let us both pray and be thankful for all the good coming our way. I am sending you my very best wishes for the holiday season as you observe it. Thank you for keeping me in your prayers. I sure can use it especially when coming from you. You are my sunshine.

Dear Sister, I must add this; in all your mail you repeatedly mention lack of time for yourself for all your objective reasons. Please go back to the letter where I emphasized the importance of taking responsibility for your life and health and how crucial the need for sleep and rest are. The changes of nutrition as well as the B3K are only part of the 'medications' you need to take, but water and sleep are the most important of all.

Please understand that if you don't take the time to rest you may fall behind in your healing process, even as far as if you have not done a thing for your health thus far.

Yours,

Yael

December 12, 2007

Dear Sister Paula,

We are so blessed and that I know for sure. On my sixty-first birthday, which was the night of the first Hanukkah Candle, on a Tuesday, which traditionally in the Judaism is blessed as a twofold good day, *Giggling Dr. Green* was out for the public – for the first time.

On December twelve of two thousand and seven, my youngest son's thirty-first birthday, and your check arrived and the first box of books arrived as well. To me it seems so symbolic having all those significant events happen at those significant dates. I appreciate your payment. Please allow me to keep it on my desk and see in it the beginning of the flow of light to many more people and children around the world. It will always remind me to stay humble and know that it is not my success, but just the guidance for me to try and help reach as many listeners as possible in order to contribute in creating a better world.

The law of giving and receiving in our universe has been materialized. You sent your gratitude my way as well as I have sent my thoughts and guidance to the universe. I am sending a copy of *Giggling Dr. Green* to you today.

May you be blessed forever with good health, inner fulfillment and inner happiness.

Love,

Yael

December 17, 2007

Dear Dr. Yael,

On Saturday I received your book *Giggling Dr. Green* in the mail, which was a very happy moment for me to actually see it and hold it in my hands. I feel very honored that you personally signed the book for me and that you included my name among those who helped and supported you in the realization of this project.

Writing a book is not easy, especially for a book like yours that carries such a powerful message to the people of today and challenges the establishments, their laws and greed. As I browse through the whole book I see that it is certainly very interesting and useful not only for children but for adults as well who will benefit of all the vast information you share. I intend to read it very thoroughly and continue and support you by making your book known to other people as much as I can. In this special season of the year when we read and remember the messages of the prophets of long ago, promising salvation and light to

234

mankind, your book appears like a beacon of light to the people of today walking in the darkness of ignorance. Your name can certainly be recognized not only as an author but also as a prophet for the present time.

May God Bless you with the abundance of His light always.

With love and prayers,

Sister Paula

December 18, 2007

My Dear Sister Paula,

I just received your wishes for my book and they are very touching and affirming to me.

I thank you for your words.

You were right when you mentioned my intention in *Giggling Dr. Green* to send a very strong message to as many children and people I possibly can, hoping to avoid the victimization by the monetary driven medical establishment of our era. I also like to draw parents' attention to the other industrial fields like TV, video games, furniture, clothing, makeup, creams, strollers, toys, processed food and harmful beverages, and many more. Those entire latter disregard the children's well-being, and care only about their lush income.

Your words of encouragement and appreciation mean the world to me especially coming from a personality as you are. I wish to get your permission to put those last paragraphs in your last email on my website so it may lead people to peek into *Giggling Dr. Green* and maybe even help save the next generations to come. I feel honored to send you my book and to stick your check to my window. I prayed to the universe many times and asked to earn my income only through good deeds for this earth's inhabitants. Your money opens the door for the distribution of this book. After all, we adults have the choice to change from ignorance to enlightenment at any given moment yet, the little babies and children depend upon those who should be trustworthy like their parents, family members, caregivers, doctors, nurses, teachers and authorities, who are harming the babies and children and whether through their ignorance or for the sake of the money, is in my opinion a hideous crime.

This is precisely my *Giggling Dr. Green* book's mission. With love and thanks I wish you all the very best.

Yours,

Yael

December 18, 2007

My dear Sister Paula,

Your words are very touching and affirming to me. I thank you for your words.

You were right when you mentioned my intention in "Giggling DR. Green" to send a very strong message to as many children and people I possibly can and hope to be able to avoid their victimization by the monetary driven medicine establishment of our era. I also like to draw parent's attention to the other industrial fields, like TV games, furniture, clothing, makeup, creams, strollers, toys, processed food and harmful beverage, and many more. Those entire latter disregard the children well-being, and care about their lushes income only. Thank you so much for sending your words of encouragement and appreciation. It means the world to me especially coming from a personality as you are. I wish to get your permission to put those last paragraphs on my web site so it may lead people to peek into *Giggling Dr. Green* and maybe even help

238

save the next generations to come. I feel honored to send you my book and to stick your check to my window. I prayed to the universe many times and ask to earn my income only through good deeds for this earth's inhabitants. Your money opens the door for the distribution of this book. After all we adults have the choice to change from ignorance to enlightenment at any given moment yet, the little babies and children depend upon those who should be trustworthy, like their parents, family members, caregivers, doctors nurses, teachers and authorities, who are harming the babies and children, whether through their ignorance or for the sake of the money, is in my opinion a hideous crime. This is my Giggling Dr. Green book's mission.

With love and thanks I wish you all the very best,
Yael

December 24, 2007

Dear Dr. Yael,

Reading your book *Giggling Dr. Green* is just like talking to you as I had the privilege to do in the past along all our many conversations. It is a wonderful learning experience for me as it clarifies so much for me. It becomes easier to understand how we all came to this world equipped with our basic wonderful, self-healing abilities, through the vast knowledge and experience you offer.

Through Johnny's letter in your prologue you carry the reader into your book with a very powerful beginning, followed by the chapters leading to the challenge, opening a new door to the suffering children who had been and still are so wrongly treated and nourished in today's society.

I presented and recommended your book to a few people, parents and doctors, yet the resistance to the natural approach unfortunately is very concerning. Your mission will make a difference in the world to those who are open and willing to accept it and assume responsibility for them and their families' well-being, rather than believe in the mainstream's magic wand. (I was surprised to see the staggering number of over 300,000 people a year who die of medication side effects, wrong medications, overdosages and unnecessary or just medications per say, wrongly diagnosed, wrong surgeries, surgeries complications etc. in the USA.) I continue to pray that this book will serve its mission to many responsible parents and family members, teachers and friends, and that God's power and strength will protect and always support you.

In regards to my health, I have been doing very well, thank God and you. I can be a living proof how the natural way of living is the best and only choice. Tomorrow, Christmas Eve and then Christmas Day, even if you do not celebrate Christmas as I do, I want to wish you a Blessed Christmas. If there is a person in the world with the true spirit of Christmas it is certainly you. Peace, love, compassion, joy, simplicity of life, this is what Jesus wanted to give the world. Now we must be His heart, His arms, His presence to a world that has forgotten why He was born among us, and this is what you are and have been for many children and people of every age along your blessed life.

May God be your comfort and your strength forever,
Sister Paula

January 13, 2008

Dear Dr. Yael,

I have not written to you since the beginning of the year. I was very busy reading your book every free moment I had. For me it has been like talking to you closely as if you were here right here sitting on the chair opposite the table facing me every day, since your book is in truth, wonderful, so refreshing, and honest with immense information, and brings all your immeasurable knowledge and experience to the reader. But even more it brings your whole self. I deeply admire you for your courage to speak so clearly against the wrongs of modern medicine and the modern world, and for revealing yourself so openly to your fellow readers. Some parts of the book are really your autobiography. *Giggling Dr. Green* is certainly a great gift to the present generation of parents and their children and families.

How was your book perceived by the community at large and in the medical circle? Do you encounter any problems due to your honest writing? I wonder and would like to tell you that I worry also because, even in my small experience, I can see how difficult it is for people, educated people as well as less enlightened people, to accept new (in reality, ancient) and or different ideas in the health and nutrition field.

Personally, I continue to follow your "living healthy" lifestyle and nutritional advice, and the B3K is now a vital part of my daily schedule. Thank God I am doing very well. You told me that I am a pioneer in taking this path under my circumstances and in my community, but I am a pioneer without followers, and sometimes I wonder for how long can I continue without being overridden by the pressure of the establishments.

However I am thinking positive and I am sure that God will always help me to follow His will, which I hope to be my self-fulfilling prophecy.

I am back to reading more of your book so I may learn some more about the homeopathic remedies and to try some of your recipes. There is so much to learn that I cannot absorb it all by reading it once. I wish you again success and the best results with your book.

Thank you for the beautiful New Year card; you are always in my prayers and my heart.

Love,
Sister Paula

January 14, 2008

Dear Sister

Presently I am in Israel and like almost everyone around me, with the flu. I forgot how bitterly cold Israel could get in the winter. The reports about people who die of the cold are alarming, especially in Israel which is known for its normally very hot weather. Unbelievable how Israel, the social democratic country, would be unable to protect the poor from hunger and cold, and not let her people, among them many concentration camps refugees, old and poor who die of it. Israel is renowned for the desert heat in the summer and the mild winters, though this year everything has changed to the deadly extreme. It is so sad to watch it on the news and not be able to do much about it mainly as a guest who is sick too like the others. I am thankful for the many charity organizations that care for the needy and do all they can in order to serve best the unfortunate and helpless members of the human community.

I feel honored and flattered to learn that you read and enjoy my book, *Giggling Dr. Green.* Thank you also for your enlightening and empowering comments. Truthfully I have so far received only similar feedback like yours, and I don't know anything about the medical community and how they feel about the book, provided they had read it at all. The surveys indicate that our health services are by far the worst health services in the entire western hemisphere and only some of our doctors open up to learn and respect the holistic medicine as they come to realize that nature's power of healing must be considered and cannot be ignored. *Giggling Dr. Green* is only one more voice claiming to stop the wrongdoing and horrific injustice done to the innocent and to the heartless torture through useless treatments and medical procedures of a whole world of children. I appreciate your e-mail and hope to always hear your true thoughts.

I pray that you will never succumb to the mainstream medicine and will only regenerate your good health by your own power. Please continue and never give up. Please don't let the ignorance and corruption kill your innocent soul and body.

With best regards,

Yael

January 27, 2008

Dear Dr. Yael,

I was sorry to hear that you were not doing so well in Israel. I really hope that by now you have improved and you can truly enjoy your visit in your homeland. Florida is cold these days too, but it is a pleasant cold causing no hardship. I like this weather; it feels as if it gives our body new energy and enables the activities outdoors to be really enjoyable. I am making little progress introducing your book to people I meet like parents and teachers who displayed great interest in it. One of my sisters, who is skeptical of my choice, is reading *Giggling Dr. Green* now but I have not gotten any comment from her as of yet. I am reading *Her-2* by Robert Bazell and have to admit that I am shocked as I read about all the suffering and deaths of so many women and the doctors' blindness in spite of all their research. I do not understand everything in that book but I cannot avoid comparing myself to those women. Here I am, living on salads, feeling well and healthy, and think; am

I free of cancer? I feel like I am even if I cannot prove it now. I try to understand why the natural approach to cancer is completely disregarded in all those scientific pharmaceutical cancer researches. (Is carrot and celery juice not making big money for the pharmaceutical industry to be that far disregarded and pushed away?) My sisters often repeatedly request to return to the mammogram now but I resist their pressure because I do not know what the results may be. Eventually I will have to do it and I hope to wait at least one year and whatever the results may be will not change my choice. I would like to hear your opinion about that, please.

In my professional life at the convent, we are expecting a few changes this week, yet nothing even close to what I was hoping for. The assistant I had is leaving Florida, so Monday I will begin to train a new person who needs to be prepared for the kind of service of the disabled young adults we provide. I will have to resume a full time schedule, which I did cut back since September of 2007. Even under those circumstances I thank God for my

250

present health and energy. Each morning when we pray from the Psalm, "O Israel, bless the Lord, Praise and exalt Him above all forever," my heart and my prayers go especially to you that God will protect you in the Land of Israel and bring you back soon to the U.S. safe and sound.

I am sending you my love and prayers—

Sister Paula

January 29, 2008

Dear Sister Paula,

Thank you; I appreciate your concern and prayers and am even happier to tell you that in spite of the bitter cold and the flu my stay in Israel was good and joyous. I met friends and besides work, spent quality time with my daughter and my grandchildren. Your prayers probably manifested in reality. I love to be in Israel—a place I feel spirituality more than any other place I visited so far. It feels to me as if I am closer to my ancient ancestors and roots. I was at the top of Mount Tabor and visited the old covenant called the "Covenant of the Silent." Since I was a young girl, probably around the age of 9, the stories about the "Covenant of the Silent" and the monks who never talk absolutely fascinated me and I was eager to see it and experience it from the inside. At the age of ten, our whole girl scouts pack went on a field trip to that same area, planning to climb up that mountain and visit the covenant. Like plans sometimes tend not to work out, this one did not work out either, and we never climbed up this mountain and never reached our goal—the "Covenant of the Silent." Five years ago, on one of my trips to Israel, I went to that mountain and accomplished that old childhood unfulfilled plan and I was fifty-six years old. It was a magnificent experience I had and this time, too.

The trail up is a pretty challenging serpentine, a partially paved road on a very narrow an utter steep path. The visibility is dangerously limited due to the steep rocky mountain and curves sight yet it would not slow the cab drivers from rushing up and down the hills almost like on our wide-open highways. Even though I am not considered to be a courageous driver, it did not scare me away from pursuing my dream, and I made it up Mount Tabor determined this time to achieve my goal. As you know I am not a religious person by any means, and do not serve and observe any religion, yet it still made me feel as if I was getting closer to God and touch history. I could almost sense the trace of the many generations of footsteps that went up that high mountain to this ancient covenant. The old olive trees along the curving serpentine trail were standing there as monuments in silence witnesses of history. Each tree in its own shape, and maybe even pride, strong and tough enough to withstand the rough weather and climate, in addition to all the wars gone past that the trees have survived. These precious trees provided men with olives, wood and shade for generations, for better nutrition, for light and heating; wood for fire, shelter and furniture, olive oil for food, soap and even medicines, and could out-weather for centuries the storms, the hot summers, the scarce water for rain is very little in Israel, the cold and harsh winters, the many wars and bloodshed in this little country—Israel. Those olive trees have seen it all.

And thus their silence reflects their strength; they continue existence and the stories they could tell. It felt as if those beautiful olive trees were there to tell me and everyone who listens to their whispers, not to fear, but continue to climb up to the mountaintop and feel how 'godliness' and 'magic' and divinity can truly feel.

The widely open view allows the viewer to see all the neighbor countries around as they walk on top of that amazing mountain. It felt mighty and so close to heaven, especially the slight caressing breeze, which felt for a moment as if the universe was tenderly embracing me and caressing my wide spread wings. It was the closest I had ever felt to divinity. No synagogue or church could bestow me this enigmatic love for me ever before. Traveling and touring that area brought me you. Isn't that a nice way to keep contact with a close friend?

This is a little ancient historical description of mount Tabor in the Bible, "Deborah sent for Barak son of Abinoam from Kedesh in Naphtali and said to him, 'The LORD, the God of Israel, commands you: 'Go, take with you ten thousand men of Naphtali and Zebulun and lead the way to Mount Tabor. I will lure Sisera, the commander of Jabin's army, with his chariots and his troops to the Kishon River and give him into your hands.'"(Judges 4:6-7)

"You created the north and the south; Tabor and Hermon sing for joy at your name" (Psalm 89:12).

"Jesus took with him Peter, James and John the brother of James, and led them up a high mountain by themselves. There he was transfigured before them. His face shone like the sun, and his clothes became as white as the light.

"Just then there appeared before them Moses and Elijah, talking with Jesus. Peter said to Jesus, 'Lord, it is good for us to be here. If you wish, I will put up three shelters—one for you, one for Moses and one for Elijah.' While he was still speaking, a bright cloud enveloped them, and a voice from the cloud said, 'This is my Son, whom I love; with him I am well pleased. Listen to him!' When the disciples heard this, they fell facedown to the ground, terrified. But Jesus came and touched them. 'Get up," he said. "Don't be afraid." When they looked up, they saw no one except Jesus. As they were coming down the mountain, Jesus instructed them, "Don't tell anyone what you have seen, until the Son of Man has been raised from the dead" (Mt 17:1-9).

I am proud of you for getting better and for how you hold strong in your decisions. See, it does not really matter whether the lump is still there or not. Cancer cells are very weak and the healthy body cells gradually consume them, as you know since the immune system regards the cancer cells as foreign proteins, once the immune system regains its strength and vital functionality. How fast the body is working is not as important as the fact that all your vital connections orchestrate as the self-healing mechanism are works efficiently. A lump can be there even if it is not active. Just as an old scar can remain and still be healed.

You seem to be 'gliding' on the right track. All healed cancers were healed by the same means you chose. Unlike burning and fighting cancer cells, the body strengthens its self-defense mechanism and builds immunity against this chaotic creation of hormones and uncontrollable cells. The DNA intelligence, which is in fact our blueprint, will then be able to identify any attempt of recurrence of this chaotic cell production and will respond promptly to protect and preserve your health and life. Whereas by treatments of chemotherapy, surgery and radiation, the body does not learn this vital life saving lesson and does not experience and train itself to restore health on its own, which could of course be one of the reasons for the relapses people endure and fear. Often we hear: "Now he was diagnosed with cancer in a different organ," and these statements are foolish. The poor person never got the chance to heal, and the 'reason' for the 'new' cancer cells was in fact never being addressed by mainstream medicine, and like a dragon grows ten more heads when you cut one head off, so does the body respond to the mainstream cancer treatments. You cannot just 'stop' cancer by chopping the head off.

Imagine a little child learning to walk and trains its brain to stabilize and balance. If we would pick him or her up every time they fell or, like the mainstream approach to cancer, if we would amputate her or his legs because they cause the child falls with each attempt to walk, would this child ever learn to walk, dance or run? By allowing our body to learn to identify the mistakenly chaotic cell development, which is called "cancer," and support the body through lifestyle modifications and corrections, we allow our health to resume normal vitality and guard us from cancer. Although cancer research suggests that cancer starts from the genes in the DNA, I strongly advocate the opposite. Those scientists are ordered and prompted to hide the truth since the pharmaceutical companies are funding them, and those interests in medication and medical procedures are for their revenue, not for your health or my own. I have the dream that one day the truth will surface and the centuries long abusive handling of innocent patients who put their trust, hope, faith and money in their 'health services' and 'specialists' will come to an end by finally having better educated patients who will not succumb to those criminal actions any longer. TV shows talk about the "advanced breakthroughs in children cancer treatments" by "discovering the cancer causing genes." Yes, hide and never disclose the fact that we all have an ocean wide inherited tendency storage in our DNA and genes and therefore each of us has a 'predisposition' and 'tendency' for different diseases as well as cancer strains. Yet, these researchers never mention in their glorified research reports that with vaccinations and over medicating of the children, the predisposition awakens and the children's bodies create cancer cells because those mandatory vaccines are nothing but another criminal act of medicine, which in fact does nothing but totally kills and wipes the immune system we were born with - totally out. With the success they claim to eradicate most of the children's diseases 'thanks' to the vaccines; in reality they created the monstrous cancer epidemic in young children called pediatric cancer of all kinds, not to mention the high blood pressure, high cholesterol, arthritis, Alzheimer's, liver cirrhosis, kidney failure and ulcers, asthma, skin diseases, diabetes, multiple sclerosis—all old people diseases in small children. I chose a good round of the chicken-pox for my children and grandchildren, nieces and nephews when they were born over cancer and all the other 'old people's diseases' at such young age.

Now, dear sister, you only need to continue and adhere to your way. Obviously you do feel healthier and stronger, so you probably are healthy as such. We all know that "God helps those who help themselves." You have learned to make your own choices. You also have learned to take a significantly larger chunk of responsibility for your life and health and have chosen to make some of the necessary changes and adjustments, at least as far as your nutrition is concerned. Getting cancer, or better to say, "creating cancer" is a process of giving up control over our own health and life. Thus, healing cancer requires us to reclaim and assume that responsibility for our health and life by making the necessary changes in life so we may flow with the trends and changes that life is taking us along. Like in your case for example, you gave up many important stages and processes in life by joining the convent at a young age and as a result, you know better than anyone else where your life experiences have taken you throughout these past fifty years. And only you know how many times you doubted your choice in the depth of your heart asking "was it right or wrong?" Clearly, you stood fast to your decisions, and refused to contemplate and succumb to any changes or modifications. Your body is the living testimony of all your needs that were never met and never granted by you—to you.

Conversely, now you have gone out of your habitual lifestyle, daringly, and allowed some of the needed changes only because you know now that it is a matter of life and death. Whether or not those changes will suffice to combat and restore your health following the long term damage to your body or not may be reflected in a couple of years. Indeed, by feeling so much better and stronger you are bearing the fruits of your efforts and adjustments to the few changes and to your decisions to take a bigger share of responsibility, and for that I hold your hand and salute you. I still hope that you will not yield to the power of ignorance and fear that work so hard to discourage you and pull you back to the "obedience and order"—not to nature but artificially established 2000 years ago. Just keep on doing what you are on your path to good health and I hope you will gain ever more strength as you go along, inner strength as well as physical strength.

Thank you again for spreading the word about *Giggling Dr. Green*, because the message is important.

Love,

Yael

February 29, 2008

Dear Dr. Yael,

Thank you for sharing with me the wonderful story of your life, the struggles and suffering of so many years, and the glorious achievements of your happiness and love. You certainly are a great example of what the trust in the power of God can bring to the human life. I had the same impression even when I was reading some of the chapters in your book in which you reveal part of your personal life. I continually thank God for knowing you and pray for you every day. May God always guide you in the fulfilling your life as well as in enriching lives of all those you touch on your journey. Thank you also for the newsletter that has been very interesting and reassuring for me since I have been using the B3K every day. I continue to do well as the season of Lent offers me many opportunities to learn and grow on my journey to God.

It has also been a month of many difficulties trials and frustrations but I regarded them all as gifts from God and did not let them disturb my inner peace and trust in God's unconditional love to me and to the entirety of humanity. Health-wise I continue to enjoy the new way of nutrition, yet, in spite of your suggestion, I did not eat any eggs because it is so hard to find a free roaming chicken unless I start to raise them myself. Per your suggestion, I am reading the John Robbins book, *May All Be Fed*, and it does convince me not to eat any food that comes from the ocean, which is so polluted worldwide. I eat daily a good variety of vegetables, fruits, legumes and seeds, and feel well nourished with good energy and good digestion. Could the little weight I continue to lose still be part of my body's cleansing process? I do have a little problem though with the swelling of my ankle. Please, if you have any suggestions they would be greatly appreciated. I thank God for my health every day and for being able to help others around me. I live a day at a time and do not let any worry about the future, life or death, disturb me.

I know that every moment of our life is in His hands.

How are you doing with your new book? I continue to introduce *Giggling Dr. Green* to many people but the results are not so great. In spite of all the available information about the danger in medications and improper nutrition people still choose to eat irresponsibly and swallow pills for every discomfort.

I find it very sad.

I am closing this email now sending you all my love and thanks.

May God bless you always with the abundance of His love.

With peace and joy,
Sister Paula

March 1, 2008

Dear Sister Paula,

Thank you for your regards and appreciation. I don't like to scratch the clouds with my nose of your complement shower. However, I am so very happy to learn that you are doing so well. Thank the Universe. Every morning on my walk watching the birds, the sky, the grass and the weeds, I simply cannot stop thanking for my bliss; this part of my life is even better than my best colorful dreams could reach. Yes, one day I will not be here anymore as my spirit will leave the body that hosts my soul on this plane, though I see no difference because I feel so blessed and grateful for the privilege to share and enjoy the beauty I have been surrounded by. The true happiness is after all, not in anything we can buy or hold, but in our ability to appreciate nature and the abundant love surrounding us, which keeps our faith and spirit strong and fulfilled. So here is the secret to measure true mental, emotional and physical health. At the end of the day we are just part of this whole creation and no one assigned us to change it or doubt it, but share, appreciate, adore and respect it all.

I am glad that you read the book, *May All Be Fed* by John Robbins, as I absolutely appreciate and agree with him. Early in my childhood I decided to consume only what God had given us to pick without having to kill any of his creatures. At the age of ten I ran into lots of trouble and arguments with my family, of course, about the 'dead creatures' I refused to eat, but it never moved me away from my decision. All it did was stimulated my curiosity to learn more and expand my education and knowledge in order to help others understand the value and reasoning behind those nutrition suggestions. When asked about my nutrition I always say: I don't eat anything that can smile or had a mother or eyes; and I am grateful for my good health, abundance of energy, and the deep sense of forgiveness that is part of the healthy and delightful path of nutrition I have chosen. Yes, had people eaten less meat there would be less greed, less aggression and significantly less illness; instead, we would probably feel more love, compassion, brotherhood and the millions who are hungry in our world would be fed well. It is that simple.

In regards to your ankle I suggest you get white clay and apply it on your ankle mixed with apple cider vinegar, one teaspoon of clay with one teaspoon of apple cider vinegar. I am positive that you can find it in the whole food store or even online. It seems as if your lymphatic drainage is a little blocked. It could be tight undergarments and could be your spine and/or pelvis; this should be checked. It could also be caused by wearing stockings that are too tight, circulation blockage in your hip joint for some reason, or even pressure in your abdomen. Long hours sitting with your students and not enough movement, as well. I could check it through the foot pressure points if you can find the time to come to my office. On the more emotional and mental levels, one of the most typical causes for a hurting ankle is the suppressed desire and need to leave, to run or flee, to go away from a situation or place we cannot take anymore, yet we feel stuck there and stay against our will and desire. Whether it is the place we reside in, our workplace or the people we live around, if our morals and oaths dictate us to stay in spite of our deep need, our body will display the pain in those parts of the body that would help us execute and fulfill our subtle longing. A prolonged suppression, just like in your case, could take even fifty years (remember how it started with your knee pain when you were so angry at your management?). Although you steer clear of your thought and would most likely never admit it even to yourself, it could still be a reasonable cause for your ankle pain. I can't tell for sure without more information or without seeing you and as I already had offered you my service, I still welcome you to take advantage of it. The same goes for female body and emotions, which are also stored in our pelvis, and if all its functions are detoured to stay lame sexually and reproductively, the body 'adjusts' to the freezing state and debilitates the circulation and vitality of this area. Nature is simple and straightforward and accepts no tricks and oppressions neither of religion nor of orders schools and any other kinds of obedience.

If we do so—we pay.

Yours forever,

Yael

May 7, 2008

Dear Dr. Yael,

It has been since March that we last corresponded but I have been thinking of you every day and follow the 'living healthy' lifestyle, which I learned from you, but have had no time to write to you.

Did you have a chance to watch the evening news? Robert Bazell presented a series of alternative medicine and the different optional ways to address cancer. Though he did not say much, it is interesting to learn how the power of the mind in the visualization therapy or other ways are suggested as valid alternative measurements to address health problems and cancer. I hope you are doing well even if certainly, busy. Healthwise, I am doing very well.

Next Sunday our catholic celebrations are going to be Pentecost Sunday to remember the beginning of the Church when the Holy Spirit came and promised by Jesus. The Spirit of God is always with us if we do not chase Him away from our heart or mind, by clogging them with material values. I share this with you since you are a living example of the power of the Spirit in my eyes. Pentecost Sunday also closes the Easter season, the season of glory, resurrection and love.

More changes in my life during this time, neither pleasant nor good, yet I still welcome them as the manifestation of God's will and as opportunities for growing closer to Him. That is what I try to do, even if it is not so easy. I leave you now with a passage from the book of Chronicle in the Bible I came across: "The Lord is with you when you are with Him, and if you seek Him, He will be present to you." (Chr. 15:2)

With love and prayer always,
Sister Paula

May 26, 2008

Dear Dr. Yael,

Thank you for sending me the beautiful presentation of Israel's 60th Anniversary. I really enjoyed listening and watching these very meaningful pictures. It was even more exciting for me when I could read it in Italian. Lately I read several articles about Israel in the Miami Herald and about three weeks ago they had a whole section about Israel's anniversary and accomplishments. It is wonderful to watch the worldwide acknowledgement and recognition of Israel's achievements, which are remarkable and superior in every aspect, yet sad that Israel cannot achieve the most important goal—peace. Let us keep hoping and praying for Israel's peace and security. We know how the impossible for leaders and politicians (and physicians) is possible for God. There is one sentence in the presentation I personally felt so true to me: "Israel is not just a country, it is a homeland." This meaning transpires even more when translated into Italian. It is a land God chose since the

274

beginning of time to reveal himself to us, a land He destined for His people, and since time as we measure it, which is certainly not as God does, Israel will eventually be able to celebrate peace and security. And every man and woman in the world will consider Israel as their country, since our Faith was born in Israel and our souls belong there as Psalm 87 says: "Babylon and Egypt I will count among those who know me; Philistia, Tyre, Ethiopia, These will be her children and Jerusalem shall be called "Mother" for all shall be her children."

I would like to thank you again for your time during my last visit. Though I noticed a little tiredness in you, you still were there for me and helped me from your generous heart without reservation. I did not even think that you could get sick. I guess that as we are mortal species no one of us is guaranteed permanent health (as I understand health) even with a "living healthy" way of nutrition. The questions you asked me at our last session made me think a lot later on when I left. You asked me what are the things that bring extra joy in my life and my answer was: "The teaching and the work with my students." Your question certainly gave me food for thought and only then I realized how the joy of my life is actually in the Lord. I worry why this answer did not pop up spontaneously? This thought took me into self-reflection to find if my prayer and life routine, as well as the tendency to become absorbed by the people I work with, did not subvert my priorities and distort my ultimate goals. You mentioned "a deep sadness" in your letter that has been dispelled, however, by your deep Faith. I think that I understand. God's consoling presence is for me, most of the time, also an unfulfilled longing. The way I understand it: Love is a decision, not a feeling, and God's love cannot be measured by what we feel but by what we give to Him with our best, truthful and honest effort. His love is everlasting and His gifts are overwhelming and that should be enough for us. Thank you for reminding me of the importance of being appreciative of God's gifts under any circumstances.

Since I saw you and followed your advice my ankle shows signs of improvement. Now I better understand why you always see the feelings, emotions, thoughts and mental state as part of our physical discomforts rather than address only the physical body when our health is out of order. Today – Memorial Day, I went swimming in the pool for the first time this year. I will enjoy the outdoors more in June and suggest to others at the convent the same. I printed the nursery rhyme from *Giggling Dr. Green* about the best six doctors and use it as my guide. Thank you again for being part of my life and for giving me so much.

May God bless you always, with love and prayers—
Sister Paula

June 2, 2008

Dear Sister Paula,

As you know, I draw so much of what you call God's love and beauty from nature and from your inspiration, as you are the only person I know who is completely and absolutely devoted to the service of God, which is a very unique quality in our extremely material oriented society. Even though we are about to lose this connection with the higher power that you can call God or nature or universe, as well as our spirituality, any minute in our daily life, you stay in Faith.

Though I must say this: I do appreciate your commitment, I am very concerned about your thinking that doesn't change in any way as you repeat "growing closer to Him," "His," "He," taking nothing into yourself. You are still totally "in his hands." Your healing is about assuming responsibility and getting closer to *you*. Do you truly believe that only "He" does everything for you, with you, to you? If so, why is "He" not taking away your lump? Why do you juice, fast or change your diet? Why do you get angry? Is "He" too busy to do the work for you? I don't understand, but more so, I see that the hardest part in people—including you—is leading them to alternate ways and opening their way of thinking to a new way—because, as I mentioned numerous times, *the old is not working for you anymore*. I respect beliefs but, fear fanaticism to the point of suicide.

I am meeting a very religious Jewish couple today and whenever we talk, the man is always so anxious and stressed out. His stress is for nothing but material reasons, he is filthy rich, and still it is me who 'guides' him back to his own scriptures and helps him retrieve his sense of hope and trust in God's ways. He is so consumed by his material fears, yet at the same time he is also observing his religious duties to the extreme—to the point that he will not touch food or drink a glass of water in my home because I don't observe the Sabbath, which makes my home not kosher according to his religious stream. That does not suit the Lord's requirements and standards—prohibiting Jewish people like himself to taste anything at my table. On the other side of the coin, as a successful businessman who is a materialistic, money hungry man, he tells me quite often about lots of small tricky maneuvers in business, which are far from being honest and fair business conduct. He pulls these tricks quietly yet in order to hide from God's eyes he keeps his perfect religious rules in front of God. Just like with many other religions, harboring dishonesty and wrongdoings, even molestations of little boys, cheating with prostitutes, embezzlements, etc. It is hard to accept these double standards and the wrongful conduct in business, in the family, or even sexual misconducts by cardinals, bishops, Rabbis, school administrators and teachers, as well as the massive killing on the other hand by the Islamic extremists in the name of the "religion of peace." (The Islamic extremists state that, "Islam is a religion of peace" and therefore terrorize the world.) Plus, all that is executed in the name of God.

Is this how God, spirituality and religion have been understood and been spread around worldwide? The proper table settings and head covers, the veils and wigs on one side, yet the corrupted conducts on the other hand? Shouldn't the religion serve only one purpose: to find closeness with the higher power and to rise to the spiritual level with the purpose of bringing hope and peace, health, abundance, mercy, compassion, charity, love and justice to the world of all living creatures and plants—God's creation? If religious observing people hide their unacceptable manners and vicious minds from the law and from God, why do they claim to be good Jews or good Christians or good Muslims? No religion preaches for the molestation of little children, killing other ethnic groups, or cheating on your friends. These are sins in all faiths. So why don't those fake religious fanatics save their time and money and free themselves of any religious service? It is a useless waste of money and time as well as dishonest misuse, and nothing but a window covering to veil their corrupted mind and lifestyle while they preach why proper conduct should be and must be part of others lives.

They do serve God in such fanatic and meticulous ways for only one reason—cowardice.

Serving God is only possible with a clean heart and clean hands, free of monetary goals and benefits or hidden sociopathic agendas. And then we don't need God. We can live happy with/in ourselves. Strangely, as I already told you, as a little girl I wanted to become a nun. When I shared this wish with my father he smiled and said, "There are no Jewish nuns my child." Today, sixty years later, you, a Catholic nun, show up in my life and make me contemplate my spiritual world even though my God's name is "the universe." Though I may bully a significant part of the observer's communities I am committed to adhere to my truth without any reservations or fear of judgment—I believe in freethinking and speech. Now I understand why faith had lead me to be born Jewish so I could never become a nun. It would never work for me as I have always been a free thinker, very rebellious and far from being submissive and obedient. I have a strong will and walk my talk. I guess my father knew it when he looked at me with a big smile as he answered my request to be a nun. Now I feel as if he processed a nicer way to tell me what he thought rather than saying, "You? A nun? When you can't obey even your father?"

This brings me back to you and your email. Yes, I am absolutely positive that when we truly wish for something, we attract it and will receive it. In the scripts we read, "ask and you shall receive," and I know it works from my own life experience. Respectfully, when your ankle health is what you wish for, ask for healing and it will heal provided you listen and follow the guidelines you may receive.

The way to receive them is by listening very attentively to the clear signs you have been sent. Only when you will stop bending the Lord's will and listen to "his" messages, rather to the "rules and orders" of your "head sister," "bishop" etc. Since they are not God, and they bend and twist truth and honesty daily, just by ignoring the nature in us, and depriving you of anything God created for you and them. For example, fresh air to touch other parts of your body than just your face, sleep deprivation, sun deprivation, emotional suppressions, freedom of speech and life, and artificial toxic food. When you ask to change it they "doubt" the importance of it for your health. Feeding the poor on Christmas Eve. All those in my understanding are bending the sheer truth that exists only in nature. The sun and the moon never lie, never cheat. The tiger eats what is healthy for him and only when it is hungry. The grass is green only when sufficient water and sunlight is available. They don't bend the truth in disregard of nature and what you consider as god. So, if you want god to help you, be honest and attentive to *His* dictations to you as a natural creature and not as a plastic monument.

Just like with the sharp back pain you mentioned, and it healed. After all our higher power, whether called God, the universe nature or self, any name you choose, is what keeps us human, spiritual and alive, and with intention and request we can heal everything and bring anything to completion as we discussed at the beginning of your healing journey when you were diagnosed with breast cancer. It was probably the first time since early childhood that you granted yourself the permission to assume responsibility for yourself (sadly, not full responsibility though, as I mentioned at the beginning of this email). And as you disregarded your congregation's doubts and disbelief, in spite all traditional concepts, your life became your foremost priority and you took the initiative to recover your health the way you felt and understood to be the right route for you. And hence your body finally forces you to listen to yourself and your own needs as it drew your attention to finally care for your health, which has been your one and only sanctuary in which your soul resides. For the first time in your seventy-four years of existence you chose to award yourself the complete attention to your nutrition, feelings, resentments, joys, likes and dislikes and gave yourself proper rest (sadly for just a short time) in order to heal and spare your life. Why won't you think about it this way and realize how the universe delegates responsibilities, yet if we fail on our 'job' we will be reminded to go back and redo it—this time right.

At this time please get in touch with the pain you still experience and ask yourself what could be the message you are trying to tell yourself? And why is your pain manifesting in that specific part of your body? By 'talking' to your body you may obtain answers waiting dormant for many years deep within you. We chose this body as the sanctuary for our soul to reside in as long as it serves the soul's purpose on this earth. I do believe so. I believe and strongly advocate in changing our way of thinking and encourage a shift to try to understand where we are in that danger and disharmony between our core beliefs and our true deep needs.

We cannot ignore our requisites or our thoughts and thus, avoiding or denying them for long will always end in tragedy. We must be conscious of our prayers and our integrity to ourselves. We cannot just do things in life when our heart and soul are not in agreement with our passion and when we are in disagreement between our beliefs and deeds. We must be aware and make the changes we need to reconcile our serenity. We are human and as such we make mistakes. Yes, when you visited me I was sick. I knew very well that the reason for my disease unfolded due to regrets for my past poor choices. I feel though, that I got a second chance to correct my errors and indeed I made the corrections and feel better.

For now I suggest you learn to talk to yourself as you talk to God, be kind, caring and responsible to yourself as you are to God, because you and God are the very same for when you serve god you in reality serve you. Learn not do things to yourself you wouldn't have done to God.

You and God deserve the same devotion, tolerance, love, service, trust, perseverance, respect and commitment at all times. You deserve them all just like your God does. You have been serving the world with great steadfastness and loyalty your entire life and continue relentlessly because those people are absolutely depended upon you. And you are dependent upon yourself as well to be responsible for your own well-being.

I know you understand what I mean.

There are conditions and situations in life that are simply unchangeable and we have to live with the way they are. However, we all can change the way we look at and see things and can modify and improve some of the living conditions surrounding us. For example, when two people are unable to separate for any given reason they can certainly set their clear boundaries; they can separate spaces, and they can communicate and aim for good understanding through healthy and constructive communication, through mutual respect and by realizing the equal rights that they both have. They can even try and create a common goal, even as little as improving their living space by making it as cozy and beautiful as possible. This may improve how they feel in the house as well as the time quality they share together and/or apart. When we don't have enough money to eat the expensive dishes we would like or are used to, we can easily learn how it doesn't take too much to grow our own little herb garden or even our own vegetables, and prepare the best and most delicious dishes we could possibly imagine. In case we live with no yard, a small porch or even bigger empty paint or construction pots can grow the best herbs and vegetables as well. If you cannot afford to dine in a restaurant, prepare your own beauty in your own space and make it your dining sanctuary. Sometimes it takes no more than one candle and one flower to turn a kitchen table into a beautiful cozy and elegant dining table. A simple pot of rice can be seasoned with one clove of garlic and a few leaves of parsley, salt and that is all. It tastes like heaven even if the wine glass is filled with water and a little lemon or apple cider vinegar. We can create our happiness wherever we are. We don't depend on anyone else do it for us, we are our own creator, designer, cook, restaurant owner, winemaker. We are all. I believe that even in a case, for example, when you break your shoulder and used to be a good swimmer, you are blessed having healthy feet to dance. This is our privilege to be able to change our point of view so we can improve any situation even when things seem just as bad as they can get.

In your life, you have told me how you find so many faults in the way the center for disabled young adults is managed; think about how these people are being fed, educated and granted a roof over their head. If you compare it to millions of disabled children and adults, or even not disabled but still people that have no food, roof or any education, you could change your attitude regarding those you critique so harshly and unforgivably. I believe that the path for better health is not just by changing our nutrition or taking different kinds of medications or even exercise, but by taking control over our life, our sense of humor, our attitude of gratitude and mostly by getting a hold of our thoughts. Like Mike Dooley says, "Thoughts become things, so make them your best thoughts."

When a decision we made ten, twenty or even fifty years ago does not suit us anymore, it is only we who have control over our mind and spirit and only *we* can make the necessary changes for the better. Just like the prisoner who committed a crime at a young age, yet matured in prison and decides instead of wasting his time behind bars, he would rather build himself up to become a better person and live a more respectful and meaningful life once he regains his freedom. He knows he can do it, exactly like each one of us can manage any change in our life if and when our old weathered past choices do not fit our present needs and growth any longer. We need no more than our clear thoughts of what and how we would like our life to change. We only need to think—better health, or think of any changes we would like to have. They will manifest in your life once we allow the past to stay in the past.

You can probably relate to my resentment to medical research of any disease, especially cancer, now. Let me put it this way, have you ever heard a guinea pig complain about her abusive and inconsiderate husband? Or did you ever hear a mouse complain about the community demands and high standards or about their high mortgage or car payments? Imagine Mickey Mouse coming to the counselor telling him how difficult his marriage is or how his wife's infidelity on top of all their drug addiction stress have kept him from sleeping at night. Funny? Maybe, yet the truth is that those small animals are tested, tortured and compared to us humans in the drug research facilities known as science cancer research centers or Alzheimer's research centers or cardio research centers, etc., and based upon those small innocent animals reactions, disease, behavior and death, the drugs are prepared to serve our illnesses.

The 'new drugs' are supposed to be good for us and heal our health challenges. The saddest part of all is – many of us continue to believe in the ability of these medications to heal our illnesses, suffering, and even save our lives. These guinea pigs and mice and even monkeys are used in science experimentation and are compared with us humankind when searching for a medical breakthrough for sleeplessness, arthritis, asthma, cancer, high blood pressure, high cholesterol and the rest of the endless list.

Most people who are diagnosed with cancer have stories to tell, as they see no possible way out of their rut. Some cancer sick people recall a past year's deep-seated trauma, car accident, death of a loved one, excess financial stress, long lasting inflammation treated with medications, job loss and others that had a damaging impact on their health equilibrium. If asked, every cancer patient can connect the physical breakdown to some extreme event in his or her life. Or even mental, emotional or environmental exposure to toxic conditions of some kind, when their health was compromised anyhow for a long time. There are of course, more reasons and different kinds of ailments but this is just one of the many examples I bring here.

Dear Sister, going back to your sisters' doubt and discouragements, let me ask you: can you please tell me how can anyone compare mouse responses to human tragic conditions? Or the way mice respond to medications or to any stimulus or food, to human's reactions? No researched results and consequences can be accurate as long as the research objective is on the physical plane only. I doubt and find it hard to believe in all the cancer triggers from outside. I don't believe that research will ever find a solution or medication for cancer as long as the research subjects will be mice, guinea pigs or people who are already at the fourth stage of cancer, whom the FDA allowed to test (as you read at the *Her2* book) or any other living creature besides the person who is afflicted by the disease itself. And utterly not as long as the goal is only the body or the organ afflicted by cancer, as mainstream medicine treats cancer sick patients according to the different organs cancer is detected in, as if it was an illness by itself. We all adapted their same language and got used to saying breast cancer, liver cancer, pancreatic cancer, etc. (strange but could it possibly be the breast's fault or the prostate's fault and therefore it is been amputated?) The pharmaceutical research and medicinal cancer industry is so enormously profitable and the revenue off the disease is so unbelievably high that any steps taken to reveal the true therapy would create an unfathomable financial disaster, even worse than any economic disaster the world has seen yet. If this were not true, then why would the AMA and FDA approve cancer therapy by the natural way, which in reality is the only true way?

Could water, carrots and celery, or chiropractic adjustments or pulse electromagnetic field therapy, homeopathy, acupuncture and reflexology, topped with healthy professional counseling of any kind, even art therapy, visualization therapy, etc. replace a multi-billion dollars industry like the cancer therapy revenues? And if they would, who would have the courage to publish it without being subjected to FDA and AMA lawsuits, and who would be willing to sit behind bars just for practicing true health rather than a mass-killing, money-making, corrupted yet legal 'cancer therapy' monster? You know very well how those who are cancer survivors in reality healed themselves in spite of the 'cancer therapy' they received. A *cancer survivor* is every person who decided to accept the message from his or her body and make fundamental changes in his or her physical, emotional, social and spiritual life.

My very best regards,

Yael

June 8, 2008

Dear Dr. Yael,

I want to thank you very much for your long letter, which indeed gave me a lot to think about. When you talk about God and how to love and serve Him, I am always amazed by the strength of your faith and by the clarity of your vision. You, a Jewish person, really possess the spirit of the Gospel, the spirit of the Good News brought by Jesus. "Religion is not a matter of eating and drinking, but of worshiping the Lord in spirit and truth, and love each other like you." Unfortunately as mankind, even in the Catholic Church, like in any other church, there is always the danger of falling into formality and hypocrisy, turning the rules and customs into the substance of Faith rather than the meaningful true human values. The world always needed and always will need prophets to lead the people away from those dangers; the words of the prophets of long ago of whom we read in the Bible are still powerful guides in our present times to those who listen. The words

296

and examples of today's prophets, people like you or like John of the Cross, who has always been my most favored guide wrote, "Love is the fulfillment of the Law," meaning, in the word 'Law,' all the body of teaching from the Old Testament. He also wrote, "At the end of our life we will be judged only by our Love."

This is what I believe and what I am trying to live every day in my weak, stumbling, imperfect way. The assessment that you do of me in your letter is accurate but is not the whole me because my dedication to God is real, even if at times slightly shaken by doubts, superficiality, or even temptations. I believe in the power of prayers and in the reality of the unconditional love of God to each of us, and this belief is always a powerful source of strength and commitment. However, believing in the power of prayer, and sometimes experiencing amazing results, does not assure us of anything, because our destiny is in the hands of God. I was taught since I was young never to pray for the particular needs of everyday life, but always to pray for the fulfillment of the Will of God. Each of us may wish that something in the daily life would be different such as situations, people, results, love or business, but we learned never to ask for them in our prayers. God's wisdom, love and care that He surrounds us by should be enough. Here, I certainly learned from you how to cope through peace and joy with the many disappointments in my life.

I am hoping that you feel better than the last time we met. You, who are a source of strength for so many people, may you be blessed with an abundance of health, peace, love and joy from the Lord. He is the only One who can give a positive sense to our life no matter what. I am doing better since you last saw me. The swelling diminished and I finished the homeopathic drops you had given me. I continue and follow all you suggested.

May God bless you and your family, with love and prayers—

Sister Paula

July 20, 2008

Dear Sister,

This is exactly my point. Even though you had learned to pray and ask for God's will only, and never ask for your daily needs, it is high time you understand how this part in the Catholic teaching has been harmful for you and all the other old-school believers. Unless, of course, you (and all of us) understand that God is also you, us, and nature. See the conflicting message is in many parts of the bible; it says, "God created men in his own image." Then why would our needs be disregarded, hushed, suppressed and pushed away? If we all are created in the image of God and taught to please God, we must understand that our needs are as important as "His Will." *His* equals *Our*—not just an imaginary God that is sitting somewhere in heaven handing down a list of his wishes, like a child would for his birthday or for Santa Claus on Christmas.

Dear Sister, sacrifice and deprivation of nuns and other believers doesn't bring us closer to God, because we cannot love when we starve, suffer and deny ourselves. A sad, hungry, deprived and tortured person will not be able to treat his sick helpless brother with love and compassion. A suffering destitute and sorrowful child grows up to be a vile, disenchanted, mistrustful and bitter person, and as such a man may not know what happiness means or how a happy functional family should look. He may find no happiness in farming his field and grow healthy fruits and vegetables for his family to thrive because deep inside him, the little child still hurts, injured and gloomy and needs to heal before he can live a healthy, happy life. Can you really give a warm, loving hug to any of your disabled children and adults you teach, to express your warm love, other than just being a strict conservative and demanding teacher?

So, dear Sister, your religion, with all my respect, should teach the value of life and love to people not just to a virtual God, gold covered church walls, and the luxurious piece of art and precious metal made statue on the cross, but like it says in the Bible: "love your neighbor like

300

thyself." And at the same time, there must be a balance. As you completely deny your needs and only serve others and God, the religious leaders appear to be solely *self*-serving.

Loving God is fundamentally misinterpreted by the Church, by the imam and by the rabbis, and should be re-evaluated, and taught differently in order to achieve a genuinely better human society along with a deeper understanding and a healthier more compassionate world at large. Why is it that the Head of the Vatican, the Pope, lives a life of corrupted filthy abundance and material fortune in his palace, yet watches from his throne high above all the hunger, poverty and misery of wars and disease for millions in the world, yet preaches for the "need to help those poor people?" It is possible only because those less fortunate are brainwashed to believe that this is how their religion is supposed to be and they believe that this is what Christianity is. Rabbis are close to the same as are the mullahs and imams. The priests live like kings as well as the pastors and the Jewish rabbis. Churches were built with funds enough to feed the hungry all over the world, heal the sick and pay for education. And the rabbi's yards don't fall short as they are always "blessed" and never know a moment of lack, neither of food nor luxurious clothing, jewelry and cars, for themselves, their families, and all those who benefit through "gray" business relationships.

The Bible emphasizes humility and diffidence, condemning material corruption. The other religions condemn the well-appointed lifestyle on account of the poor and unfortunate as well; yet, the common people see, accept and support the church, no questions asked. Is this what "serving God" is all about? Is the imam, mullah, rabbi, priest, cardinal or Pope God? No. They are ordinary people just like you and I, dear Sister, yet live a lifestyle you shy away from even in your wildest dreams. Is this moral? Isn't it like stating, "Don't do what I do, do as I preach?" Is not the Pope surrounded by anything less than a king, yet preaches to pray only for God's will and not for your own needs? Did he? Did God put him there on his throne rather than the Church politicians and your religion's hierarchy?

The way I understand the world, this also must undergo major changes and I feel that it will this century. As I am rewriting this part, Neptune, the planet of religion and humility, as well as the planet of confusion and deception, is just entering its home sign, Pisces and for the past few months Uranus entered Aries. Pluto entered Capricorn at the end of 2008. The world is undergoing robust changes and transformations that it has not seen for centuries. This will probably change the religious world as well, globally speaking. As Neptune may "melt" global collective subconscious errors and beliefs of both Christianity and Islam, which are ruled by the same sign, they will experience the deepest transformation since about 170 years ago when Neptune was in Pisces last.

Uranus prepares the ground for this conscious melt down through the massive demonstration and standoff in what is called the Arab Spring. The Arab Spring opens the door to countless more revolutionary acts of the younger, enthusiastic, scholastic generations who demand equal rights, democracy, and who demand to put an end to the ruthless corrupt dictatorships as known mainly in the Arab and Islamic world. Islam is facing a huge change as well as Catholicism and Christianity, to adjure the era of groundless righteousness on the surface, forcing the poorly educated to believe in the power and anger of God.

Dear Sister, here is my point—in order to truly find the medicine and heal we must let go of old teachings and beliefs and reevaluate, separate the shaft from the stalk, the good and truthful teachings we grew up on from the illusionary misleading and deceiving things we observed throughout our infancy. Stunning, but worth giving it a thought.

When I first came to the USA after I was a graduate of the Israeli schools and with at least one hour of Bible studies daily, for the first time I met Christians in my daily life and was in awe as I learned the Bible's different interpretations. So different from the way I was taught throughout my entire school years and how I had assumed that all I learned was the one and only truth. The exact same psalms were interpreted completely differently from the way I was taught. The biggest shock for me was when the Rabbi said to me, "The Bible is a big book, which allows everyone to understand it the way they choose. There is no right or wrong."

I felt deeply devastated, disappointed and even betrayed. I thought, *How can anyone doubt the only right way the Bible is been understood by us, Jews, and dare to understand "our" holy book differently?* But, I had to open up my eyes and heart allowing the differences to prevail. I had to undergo and succumb to that immense adjustment in a totally unfamiliar world: religions, philosophies, rules, customs, and at the same time, embrace my evolution and inner growth. And this is my message for you too. Who says that what you have learned at the beginning of your way is necessarily the right way to understand the Bible?

It is now the 21st century, and in order to change the world to the better we must first change the immediate and smaller world, which is ourselves. In the Bible it say, "As in the macro so in the micro, and as above so below." Each one of us is the reflection of the whole world, and when we modify ourselves we do so to the whole world. The old schools are not necessarily the complete, absolute and the only right schools. It is time to rethink, and try to understand the other side of the coin.

Cancer is one of those diseases people get when they cannot take changes, cannot adjust but rather stay stuck in the place they were and are, even if it may cost them their life.

I am sending you my love and support on your journey—

Yael

July 29, 2008

Dear Dr. Yael,

It has been a long time since I wrote to you. These have been very busy days not only working but also being away from home for a brief vacation. Yet, you are coming along with me, no matter where I am, in the special place I save for you in my heart. During my vacation, as I was checking my mail on a public computer in the library, I found your e-card. A pleasant surprise which brightened my day and I thank you again! I was walking miles on the beach daily, living close to nature and God through readings and prayer. Now I am back to my routine, interrupted only by some funerals. I am so sad to watch how so many people die of cancer. My students' parents, people my age or younger, and it is so difficult to have people listen or even consider the alternative healing arts or way of healthy living, without chemotherapy or medications. I faithfully continue my good nutrition you taught me, incorporating the B3K in my busy daily schedule.

I was delighted to read your newsletter loaded with good news. Last Sunday I went to the farmers market on the beach looking for anything and everything I need. I also tried your cabbage salad, which is delicious indeed. Thank you for this wonderful letter which provides not only all the vital information, but gives this so badly needed assurance and enthusiasm for living, for the transpiring faith in the gift of life. I am also very happy about the success of your son as a reflexology technician, which certainly is your success as well. I hope that you are doing well, and your guidance and strength you give to so many of us, the Lord gives you a hundred fold of his good energy and inner peace, love and happiness.

Now I would like to share with you something dark. In spite of all the beautiful opportunities I have in my life there have been moments of great darkness. Growing older does not guarantee the consistent effort and commitment to search for the holiness and for union with God, which is the purpose of my life. I had severe abdominal pain and diarrhea, which I contribute to these dark moments. I have been going through this darkness of my soul lately and it is needless to mention how it influences my health as well. Now it is over and I am completely free of it with the help of the apple cider vinegar, the Stevia and ginger you have suggested, but especially with the help of God. Reading of the scripture and praying gave me comfort even at the time of this awful darkness. Remembering all your suggestions and advice and following them helped me to snap out of my misery after only a couple of days. Those moments of darkness and doubts reveal to me how fragile I really am and how desperately I still need to grow in my faith and love to God and return to my doubtless, blind ability to follow and accept his might. Please pray for me that after all I received from his goodness I will never doubt my faith in him again and never be unworthy in reaching His Kingdom.

With love and prayers,

Sister Paula

August 1, 2008

Dear Sister Paula,

Intuitively I knew you were doing well and yet, I was thinking of you. After all, the saying goes, "No news, is good news." I send my daily gratitude for my privilege to be of help to those who truly want to change their life habits and who are willing to find true, deep, inner, long lasting, good health with a peaceful mind. To be "part of your luggage" on all your trips allows me to take part in your beautiful vacations; nice long walks along the beach in nature and all that without moving a finger. I can join you in chapel and ride the wave of all prayers, gratefulness and spiritual energy. I always loved, as you already know, the architectural interior designs of chapels here in the United States, in Europe and Israel. For some reason the feeling centuries back visitors like me had left their spiritual marks and being there all by myself made my heart feel closer to my ancestors and divinity as if they were just an arm length away. The Gospel music the chorus and the organ do

310

touch my sensitive heart as in concert with the smell of old, thick walls and the aged wood and the amazing art work in the window decorations. This is how I was feeling when I visited the old churches in Europe and on Carmel Mountain in Haifa at Stella Maris in Israel, and as I already described to you my visit at the Tabor Mountain monastery.

Try to be thankful to your last abdominal episode of pain and diarrhea. Those are good signs indicating your body protects you and fights for your life, regardless of whether or not it is bacteria, virus, fungi or toxic emotions. When anything unwanted enters your body or mind, your body responds. This indicates your immune system is active and responsive. Be grateful, for it is our true lifesaver, especially when instead of reaching out to an anti-diarrhea medicine you just used the apple cider vinegar and the B3K technology. I do the very same when I get sick. Since I never and under no circumstances would interfere with my system's reaction to any invasive agent, regardless what it is, I on no account would take any medicine to suppress what the body needs to expel, physically or emotionally.

So, I am very proud of you.

Your sadness about those deaths around you is understandable and very natural, yet, the sad truth is, and people don't dare taking the path to improve their health like you, even though chemotherapy and surgery do not help them heal. Since the war on cancer began with the National Cancer Act of 1971 we still see "runs for cancer," cancer research centers, fundraising avenues of numerous kinds for the 'invincible' cancer research, the fear of cancer, books about and from cancer survivors, etc. Never can any chemical substance aimed to kill or eradicate a living particle in our body (like cancer cells or virus or fungus) help restore good health. Only life can help to restore life and good health. Only LIFE can heal and create LIFE. Cancer, fungus of all kinds, are not in the acute disease territory of the body, but in the territory of long time suppressed acute diseases and /or disorders. Any additional cancer suppression or killings will be just a temporary

312

illusionary relief for the patient and significant revenue for the medical service industry, and no healing is taking place, regardless what the tests indicate. The body's reason for allowing cancer to settle has not been addressed and the body will simply settle those same cancer cells in a different part of its being. This is precisely the meaning of the so commonly used doctors verdict, "Sorry, there is nothing we can do for you anymore, your cancer metastasized to your _____." Fill in the blank.

I experienced that same sadness and frustration too often, up until I realized how we were all born equal and with the same opportunities and guidance. The only differences are the choices we make along our path of life. The vast health promoting and guiding information is out there for everyone who reaches out for it.

Personally I do respect those with all their different choices, and always see it as the choice of their soul. I also see in death the end of the spirit's mission for this lifetime, since I do believe in reincarnation, and in the soul's choice into which body to manifest this time on this planet. Not

313

everyone agrees with me, of course, yet this is how I see life and death and our different preferences to accomplish what we originally came here for.

Please do not worry about the energy and light I am spending so generously and share with so many people. As you probably know there is no real vacuum on our planet, emptiness will soon fill with more energy. Like in classes or in any working area when a chair in class remains unoccupied, it will soon be found by someone else who needs it. When a teacher is absent, a substitute teacher will replace him before long. When air flows out of the lungs it will be replaced by new fresh air right away. Water runs into any open space unless there are good levies. So it is with energy, generosity, kindness, light and love, mercy and compassion. The more you give, the more you receive in return from everywhere. When people can't afford my services they still will receive my help and not withstanding, I never lack anything I possibly need. All I need is always there at my disposal, be it love, abundance, energy, generosity light, a roof over my head, help, healthy food—and the universal care.

I can sense the renewed power in you. You and I are not getting old; we mature. Like good wine, the older the better. Please keep in mind the more you experience in your life, the higher your soul evolves and the community you serve and belong to, rejoice. Now I have a very serious and important question to you. I saved our e-mail exchange because there are so many significant and precious gems in them, which could be important for the whole world to read. You and I exchanged love, help, warmth, care, respect and tolerance, holiness, spirituality, health advice and knowledge I assume many more people could find helpful had they been with us and had they listened or read our thoughts and feelings. Could I please get your permission to add those letters into my new book? You are aware of my intentions as being helpful to as many people as I could possibly reach. And secondly, shall I use your name or just your initials? I will await your reply and in the mean time, I am sending you love, appreciation, thanks, and respect for who you are.

Thank you for all your help, love, prayers, enlightenments and presents.

Yours,

Yael

August 7 2008

Dear Dr. Yael,

I am so grateful for your last email. It reassured me that I am walking the right way. 3I feel very well and received a clean bill of health at my recent checkup. The doctor couldn't believe my tests results and maybe his professional pride did not let him congratulate me.

I respect his feelings and did not talk with him about the way I chose. I don't think he was ready to hear it. Thank you so much for all your patience and support you gave me all this long time of healing, and you never showed me any reluctance to answer all my doubts. Even my sisters expressed their appreciation. I never showed them any of your email, because your critique was a little harsh at times.

Now to your question about our email exchange. Dear Dr. Yael, I don't have anything to hide, my English is not a literature English, but if the content could save even one person, I feel very honored to be part of your new book. In regards to my name, I also have no need to hide, and in fact I like it to be honest all the way. So, yes, thank you for the honor, and of course you have my permission to publish our email exchange. Thank you, thank you, thank you.

May God bless you with his love and health for all the good and kind help you give His sheep.

Love

Sister Paula

Reflections

I wish that this story had a happier ending. Sister Paula did eventually get a clean bill of health, but she never fully embraced her potential with homeopathic healing. She was afraid to truly commit to her health, and found the homeopathic diet and lifestyle too inconvenient. I suspect that even after recovering her health she is not really a believer in the process and will suffer far greater at the hands of doctors if the cancer returns. Peer pressure is so powerful that people choose chemotherapy rather than abstaining from eating and drinking the poisons that helped cause the cancer in the first place. People choose to destroy their bodies in the name of treatment rather than nurturing their bodies so they can live a healthy life.

I hate seeing people die of cancer, especially knowing that the body is powerful enough to protect itself—we just weaken the body with out lifestyle.

Epilogue

Sister Paula was doing well regarding her breast cancer and continued serving and exercising her hard work at the center for mentally and physically challenged adults. She declined any mainstream recommendations of any sort and was still praying that more people would have the courage to fight for their health instead of fighting cancer. However, as we all know how hard and uncomfortable is changing our habits, and long walked paths of life, beliefs, and convictions. Men are known for finding it even harder than women when they are asked to alter their culinary customs or reconsider their state of mind, daring to rethink, or think out of the box by letting go of old beliefs. We will heal only when we understand only by changing our outlook and the way we perceive social and peer pressure. Sister Paula soon regressed back to her old lifestyle and old beliefs, succumbing to the same pressures as before she fell ill, working too hard for her age and enduring severe sleep deprivation. Sister Paula fell ill again a few years after enjoying good health, yet resented the changes she knew she had to make to remain healthy and live. As she mentioned in our email exchange more than once that she could not see her life worthy to be lived without her work. This happens to many of us when people get older and fear retirement as we dread the feeling of uselessness. This was Sister Paula's fear. After a six healthy years, she called me upset and disappointed that she was sick and felt no strength in her body to overcome her illness anymore. As indicated throughout her emails, Sister Paula never assumed complete responsibility for her well-being, as well as for her health and contentment, and left it all to Jesus, worked beyond her capacity, took no time to eat and sleep and broke down at the age 80. Sister Paula never found an hour in her busy schedule to visit my office for my treatments, in spite of her fear of death. All she could assume for a while was a better diet and trying to be less angry, which were as far as she would make any changes in her life. It was absolutely impossible for me to pull her out of her tight cling to her five decades of absolute commitment to her vow. Nothing could move her, even though she was sure that she made big changes, but she had not truly changed. Sister Paula's changes never reached her core, but her diet and pulse electromagnetic therapy only. Her lifestyle was still of hardship and absolute selflessness, and handled by the outer world rather her own inner world, which should be considered legitimate in her age without being judged as selfish.

The most important lesson we all must know by now is this: *When we walk the same path, we will arrive at the same destination.* We cannot keep on doing the same things we had done before and heal. We create the cancer cells at the time when our being (not just our body) reaches a point of desperation and resigns. As confusion in its biological equilibrium and loss of control over its own vital functions (most cancer cases pride themselves of their perfect control over their business, class, community, etc. but look at their own life "hanging" somewhere in the distance) and its ability to cultivate and replenish its own life force, which happens not necessarily just due to physical injury of any kind, not by smoking or from secondhand smoke, or by water, color, air, dishes, or our daily world surrounding us necessarily, but more often by disability to deal with their own life, harboring negative emotions and harmful experiences rather than releasing that toxicity in a constructive and healing way.

For example, my husband sees my son's shop and is upset of how untidy it is, and his own office and surrounding is dirty and messy. He would be insulted if anyone would draw his attention to it.

Sister Paula saw "all the people who are unwilling to assume responsibility for their health and learn from my book, *Giggling Dr. Green*," and yet did not realize how she was not making the necessary changes and failing to assume that same responsibility.

Hence, if we don't initiate the necessary change—change will happen anyway, but it will be painful and uninvited. Water becomes stagnant unless it is moving, flowing, and changing. Our immune system's ability or disability to function is greatly dependent upon our social

323

skills and adjustability to life and environment not any less than by what we eat and drink. When thinking of how downbeat feelings and an unenthusiastic mindset can make us sick, on the other hand we say, "laughter is good for your health" as fear creates all sorts of biochemical reactions in the body, like high blood pressure, clammy hands, dry mouth, palpitations, cold shivers, high cholesterol and irritable bowels. People always tell me, "After that accident…" or "With that loss…" or "It was a horrible shock…" and "I could not move for weeks…" and "This was when I first got sick." And they are right. Our body secretes the hormones that are so vitally needed at times of danger and harsh conditions. Every calamity, unpleasant surprise, loss or attack on us that is too hard to deal with will do the trick. These hormones such as epinephrine, norepinephrine, dopamine, phenylalanine, tyrosine, though necessary to reinforce the blood supply to the heart and muscles when under any threat or danger, turn to be very toxic after the danger is over and the body must neutralize them in order to get them out of the system once they are not needed anymore. In our reality, our physiology responds the same way regularly in our daily life due to stress and our life conditions we allow to distance and alienate us from nature. We always live in stress and anxiety. There for those same rules apply for negative thoughts; if this is your normal way of thinking, living, working, and interacting, you better become aware of this tendency and at the same time, your body routinely creates these toxic secretions. Changing the way we perceive our environment and our reactions and interaction, our responses and self-control are of vital importance and even critical in the art of cancer prevention and healing and many other terminal and degenerative diseases. Notice the same goes for the our interaction with nature, as exposure to the sun light, the fresh air, open space, water, mountains, outdoors, etc.

All those critical life conditions challenge and deprive our health, so we turn to be like a sun and water deprived plant. Sister Paula could not integrate into her orderly, strict, merciless, conservative and harsh lifestyle, and she sadly succumbed to the consequences. Had Sister Paula be able to make real changes in her lifestyle as was necessary for her full recovery, she would allow fresh energy into her being.

Sister Paula was an important mentor for me as I learned how strong the religious fear and brainwashing still holds fast in people who grew up in an extreme orthodox upbringing. She reflected to me how hard change is for us, even when looking directly into the eyes of death. We know how difficult the withdrawal of any addiction is, so are the deep-seated habits, beliefs, and convictions. It is not less difficult to change when at an older age we wake up from our childish illusions and see all the wrongs, injustice, misuse and corruption of the governing instances, and realize that "the king is naked." I mean that we were led to believe but it is not true and should not be part of our belief system. We are afraid of the doctors' warnings because we have too much confidence in the doctor's education and experience. We still fall into those dogmas and just a few of us question the obvious.

Sister Paula made me happy, sad, angry, frustrated, and confused throughout our encounter because I often felt as if I was running against a brick wall. She cultivated my tolerance to those who are so radically different from me. I guess it was not only me sent to her to save her life, but she was sent to me to save my understanding. Had Sister Paula be able to make real changes in her lifestyle as was necessary for her full recovery, she would allow fresh energy into her being.

I often mention energy flow because this is what change is all about. As the moon and the sun radiate their energy and enable existence, and the inhaling fresh air interchanging with exhaling impure and used air is life, so must the old energy give way to the new energy. We accept those changes in our daily life as a must, and as a given. Though for some of us even to throw the unnecessary, old and used out, most of us know—throw out the old and make room for new. This is just like energy flow in every realm in our life. We watch the ebb and flow of the oceans, seasons change, and trees change colors. So must we change for our life.

Along the years of practice I found how hard the change of life habits has been to most people.

Never the less I like to bring just a few names and Cancer cases who successfully made the needed changes and never had a recurrence of cancer.

Don 67- Florida was diagnosed with "aggressive" colon cancer. He was operated yet one month later it just got worse. He asked me for help and after seven years told me how he was kicked out of his doctors office because he was completely well. He continued to follow a healthy lifestyle.

Nava 32 - Israel, was diagnosed with malignant Leukemia healed. 17 years later I heard from her and about her good health.

Rina 56- Israel, had a 20 cm tumor in her back, after 2 months, was declared clean.

Janet 45- Colorado, came to me with fourth stage bone cancer on a wheelchair, after three month was clean of cancer.

Jay 44- Oregon. Leukemia recovered.

Petrick 73 - NJ. Fourth stage cancer of his skin. Recovered and still is.

Dmitry 28 - Ca. Called me when he had 6 more weeks, yet refused chemo and followed my suggestions. 5 months later he called with his exciting news that he just received his tests results and was clean and got married.

Ariela 57 - Israel- Brain tumor. Healed and still works 7 years later.

Sharon 13 - Israel, brain tumor. Recovered her blindness and resumed her school.

Adi 6 - Neuroblastoma. Had 5 more weeks to live according to the doctors, healed and resumed normal life after just 2 months.

And the list goes on.

THE END